GLUTEN-FREE BREAD

for Beginners

EASY AND DELICIOUS GLUTEN-FREE BREAD RECIPES

SHASTA PRESS

ISBN: Print 978-1-62315-212-3 | eBook 978-1-62315-213-0

CONTENTS

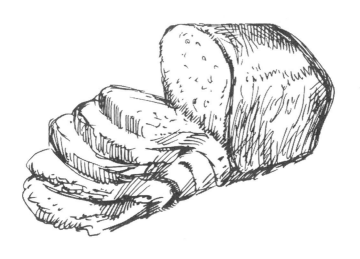

*How can a nation be great if its
bread tastes like Kleenex?*

—Julia Child

INTRODUCTION

Gluten-free diets are not just the latest fad. Ever-increasing numbers of people are choosing to embrace a gluten-free lifestyle as awareness of celiac disease, wheat allergies, and gluten intolerance grows. Whether you have decided to live gluten-free by necessity or by choice, following a gluten-free diet can be a challenge. It is a lifestyle change that requires diligence, creativity, and a commitment that will help you get past the daily hurdles.

Gluten-Free Bread is designed to help you make the transition to gluten-free bread with less confusion and more delicious recipes. This book will explain what gluten is, the different health issues people may have with gluten, and how to live without it and still enjoy great breads and treats.

It's important that you make your gluten-free decision an informed one. If you feel your body reacts badly to gluten or to wheat products, it is essential to be tested for celiac disease before you cut gluten from your diet. This test diagnoses the disease by looking for specific antibodies, which will not be present if you are no longer eating gluten. That's why you must take the test *before* you change your diet.

It is essential to understand the exact reason why your body doesn't tolerate gluten because there are important differences between celiac disease, wheat allergy, and gluten sensitivity. It's also the only way you'll know if other family members are affected, since celiac disease tends to be inherited. Once you know why your health is affected by eating gluten or wheat, you'll know how seriously you need to take going gluten-free, whether your problem is all types of gluten or just wheat, and whether deviating from the gluten-free diet is a matter of choice or a matter of safety and health.

What Is Gluten?

Gluten is a compound protein that, along with starch, is stored in the endosperm of certain grassy grains, such as wheat, barley, rye, and spelt. The endosperm is the part of a seed that stores food for the developing plant embryo. In bread, the gluten creates a crisscross protein network, which in turn, gives the dough its elasticity. This network also traps gas, which helps the dough rise. It's the gluten that gives bread its chewy texture and specific look and feel.

When you decide to eat a gluten-free diet, it suddenly seems that gluten is in everything—and it is in a great deal of things you might not expect. It can be difficult at first to weed out all of the foods you're used to eating but can no longer have. Fortunately, there are plenty of ways to enjoy many of your favorite foods by using recipes that take traditional favorites and make them without wheat, barley, rye, or spelt. There are many wonderful recipes in the cookbook section of this book, and even a bonus selection of gluten-free treats you may have thought you'd have to do without, such as pizza and even French bread.

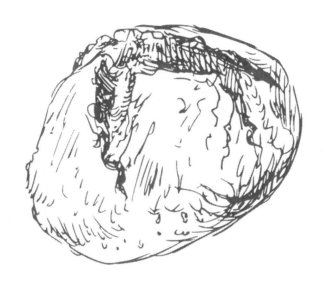

If thou tasteth a crust of bread,
thou tasteth all the stars and all
the heavens.

—Robert Browning

1

15 STRATEGIES FOR BETTER GLUTEN-FREE BREADS

You can definitely create gorgeous loaves of gluten-free bread if you follow the recipes carefully and keep these strategies in mind. You must also remember that gluten-free breads will be different from traditional wheat breads. Here are a few things to consider when baking gluten-free breads so that the experience is satisfying and successful.

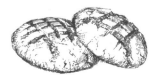

#1 Remember that gluten-free breads are definitely not like traditional breads, either in texture, taste, or even shelf life. Don't despair though—you will still be able to slice it for sandwiches, dip it in soups, and have it as toast in the morning. Some gluten-free breads are actually quick breads, so expect a certain denseness and lack of crust. Try to embrace the unique qualities of these breads without comparing them to their wheat-based counterparts. You will be able to produce some truly delicious breads that are healthy. But as with regular baking, not every attempt will be a success the first time around. Be willing to adjust and experiment to get the results you want.

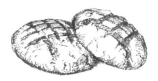

#2 If you are making yeast breads, make sure your ingredients are at room temperature, unless otherwise specified in the recipe. Yeast needs a warm environment to rise, so it is important to give it a head start, especially without the properties of gluten to help this process along. Many gluten-free flours are stored in the refrigerator. So, to get the best results, take the time to set them out before starting to make your bread.

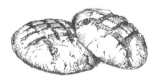

#3   Make sure you measure your ingredients carefully. Gluten-free baking is not the time to throw in handfuls and dashes except perhaps with the spices or herbs. Measure your dry goods using the spoon-and-level method, which is when you spoon the flours into the measuring cup (as opposed to scooping from the bag), and then run the flat edge of a butter knife or pastry scraper across the top of the measuring cup. This creates precise amounts of the ingredient, which can be crucial to success.

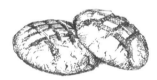

#4   Look for bread recipes that use natural leavening agents, which are what help provide volume and the needed lift to breads. Recipes that use eggs, beer, or even carbonated water will have a more traditional texture normally associated with wheat-based breads. Keep in mind also that gluten-free bread dough will look different from wheat-based breads. The dough usually will not form a ball or have the pleasing elasticity found in traditional bread making. Gluten-free dough will often look like thick pudding instead.

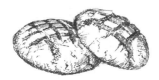

#5 Use different ingredients to create more successful finished breads. Sometimes the addition of another ingredient, even when not called for, can make your breads even better. For example, a teaspoon of pectin can be added to breads with fruit in them to give the bread a longer shelf life and more volume. As little as ⅛ teaspoon of powdered ascorbic acid (vitamin C) added to the dry ingredients in yeast breads can promote increased volume because yeast likes an acidic environment.

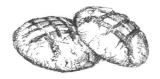

#6 Invest in some high-quality kitchen equipment such as a heavy-duty mixer because some breads need to be beaten. Also, buy a quality digital thermometer to make sure the water is the right temperature for yeast growth and that the internal temperature of your finished loaves are perfect. Great bread usually has an internal temperature between 206 and 210 degrees F. In this range, the bread will not be dried out or soggy. Also make sure your oven temperature is accurate, because even 10 degrees F in either direction can make a huge difference in the finished loaf.

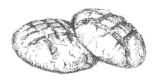

#7   If you have a drafty kitchen not conducive to bread rising, try creating a perfect environment in your oven. Turn your oven on to about 200 degrees F, and then turn it off again when it reaches temperature. Place a pan of hot water on the bottom oven rack and place the dough in the oven. This method will ensure the dough rises; however, it can cut time off the whole process, so make sure you keep a close eye on the pan. You don't want your bread to rise too much.

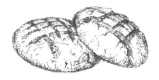

#8   Use gluten-free flours that contain more protein, whenever possible. Protein creates structure in bread, which is logical when you consider that gluten is a protein. Some great higher-protein flours to use include teff, millet, nut flours, buckwheat, quinoa, and sorghum.

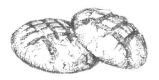

#9   Nut flours can be the base of some gluten-free bread recipes,
so it is important to be familiar with how they react during
the baking process. If you want a finer textured bread, take
the time to grind your nuts very well. If you buy ground
nut products, pulse them in a food processor to grind the
product more. The finer the nuts, the better the breads will
turn out. Also, since the consistency of the batter will be
thicker than wheat-based recipes, you will need to smooth
it out, rather than pour it into the pan. Nut flours can burn
easily, so keep your oven temperature low, no higher than
350 degrees F. Always watch the bread while it is baking
to avoid burning. If the top of your bread looks like it is
browning too quickly, cover it with a piece of foil until the
loaf is cooked through.

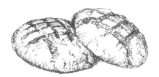

#10   Remember that coconut flour does not behave like wheat
flour. It is clumpy, dry, and unbelievably absorbent. You
will need very little coconut flour in any recipe to produce
a lovely result. You must make sure, however, to beat this
flour into your batter very well and then let it sit for a few
minutes to gauge the thickness of the batter. Since this
flour is so dry, you will need to add lots of eggs, mashed

bananas, or other liquids to offset this effect. However, if you use too much of the wet ingredients, your finished bread will be soggy and heavy. Baking with coconut flour can be a steep learning curve, but when you do master this ingredient, the results will be well worth the effort.

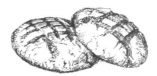

#11   Yeast can be used in gluten-free baking even though it does not create exactly the same type of rise without the gluten. The active yeast used in baking is closely related to the beneficial yeast found in fermented foods, so it can be included without adverse health reactions. You must make sure to pay particularly close attention to temperature so you don't kill the yeast organisms.

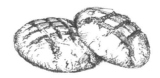

#12   Some of the products used to make gluten-free breads, such as coconut and almond flours, are expensive. If you are going to make a lot of breads and baked products, try to get your ingredients in bulk to save money. Nut flours can be stored in the fridge or freezer with no ill effects as long as they are sealed well.

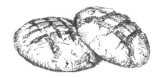

#13   Guar and xanthan gums help create rise and texture in gluten-free breads. In addition to trapping air in baked goods and making them rise well, gluten also acts as a binding and emulsifying agent. In other words, it helps hold together and even disperse all the ingredients in a batter or dough. Therefore, when you remove gluten, your end product may be crumbly or grainy. A good way to help with this problem is to add 1 teaspoon of guar gum or xanthan gum per cup of gluten-free flour. (Don't add xanthan gum to your recipe if the gluten-free flour you're using already contains it.) This helps with binding and will produce a smoother texture. Measure carefully though, because if you use too much, the end product may turn out heavy or gummy.

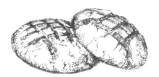

#14   Gluten-free breads can often have strange, hard crusts, which make eating and slicing them difficult. You can eliminate those crusts by placing a pan of ice or cold water on the bottom rack of the oven while baking the breads.

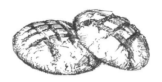

#15   Gluten-free bread does not stay moist for as long as its gluten-based cousins, so if you are not going to eat it all right away, take steps to avoid wastage. This means cooling your loaves completely, slicing them, and freezing them in resealable freezer bags. Then simply take out the slices you need and keep the rest frozen. If not freezing, most breads can be stored in an airtight container or in plastic wrap for up to three days.

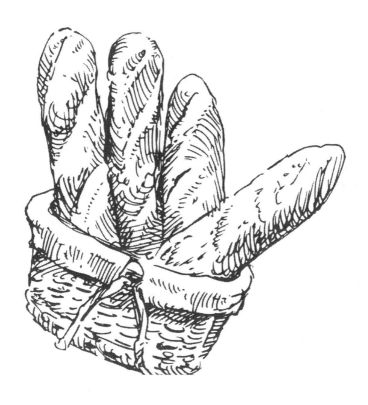

All sorrows are less with bread.

—Miguel de Cervantes

2

SAVORY BREADS

Sunflower and Quinoa Bread

This is a hearty, slightly chewy bread that is perfect for toasting because the bumps and crevices created by the sunflower seeds catch all the butter and toppings. Quinoa imparts a lovely nutty taste, which is complemented by a touch of brown sugar sweetness. Quinoa is often thought to be a grain, but it is actually a seed that acts like a grain in salads, casseroles, side dishes, and of course, breads.

- ½ cup warm water (110–115 degrees F)
- 2 tablespoons honey
- 2 tablespoons active dry yeast
- 1 cup coarsely ground raw sunflower seeds
- 1⅓ cups sorghum flour
- ¾ cup quinoa flour
- ½ cup potato starch
- ½ cup ground flaxseeds
- 2½ teaspoons xanthan gum
- 2 large eggs
- 1 cup warm water
- 2 tablespoons brown sugar
- ¼ cup melted butter
- Coconut oil to grease loaf pan

1. Lightly grease a 9 x 5–inch loaf pan and set aside.

2. In a small bowl, combine the warm water and honey, and then sprinkle the yeast on top. Let the mixture sit for about 8–10 minutes, until the yeast starts to foam.

3. In a large bowl, mix together the ground sunflower seeds, sorghum flour, quinoa flour, potato starch, flaxseeds, and xanthan gum until combined.

4. In a small bowl, whisk together the eggs, water, brown sugar, and melted butter, and add to the dry ingredients.

5. Add in the yeast mixture, mixing well for 4–5 minutes, until dough is very well combined.

6. Transfer the bread dough to the prepared loaf pan and smooth out the top.

7. Let rise in a warm spot for 40–45 minutes.

8. Preheat oven to 350 degrees F.

9. Bake bread for 40–45 minutes, or until golden and a knife inserted in the center comes out clean.

10. Let the loaf cool for 10 minutes. Then turn it out onto a wire rack until completely cool.

Makes 1 standard loaf (8–10 slices).

Crusty Boule Bread

Boule is the French word for "ball" and it simply refers to the actual shape of the loaf. For this recipe, however, the loaf looks more like a squashed ball. If you like crusty bread with a chewy texture, this will be your new favorite recipe.

- 1 cup brown rice flour
- ¾ cup sorghum flour
- 1½ cups tapioca flour
- 1 tablespoon active dry yeast
- 1 tablespoon xanthan gum
- 1 teaspoon sea salt
- 1⅓ cups lukewarm water
- 2 large eggs
- 3 tablespoons extra-virgin olive oil, plus extra to grease cookie sheet
- 1 tablespoon honey

1. In a large bowl or in a heavy-duty mixer with a paddle attachment, combine the flours, yeast, xanthan gum, and salt until well mixed.

2. In a small bowl, blend together the water, eggs, oil, and honey.

3. Add the wet ingredients to the dry ingredients, and mix until well combined.

4. Place a clean kitchen towel over the bowl, and set in a warm place until the dough rises, about 2 hours.

5. Place the covered dough in the refrigerator for up to 24 hours, or bake your bread right away.

6. Place a sheet of parchment paper on a cookie sheet and lightly grease the paper. Set aside.

7. Separate the dough into two equal portions and with dampened hands (so the dough doesn't stick), shape each into a ball. Place these on the cookie sheet with some room between the loaves.

8. Cover the dough balls loosely with plastic wrap, and let sit for 45–90 minutes to let rise again.

9. Preheat oven to 450 degrees F.

10. Using a sharp, serrated knife, make slashes in parallel lines along the top of the loaves.

11. Bake the bread for about 35–40 minutes, or until the loaves are golden. About two-thirds of the way through the bake time, set the loaves directly on the oven rack without the cookie sheet or parchment.

12. Remove the loaves from the oven and allow to cool before slicing.

Makes 2 one-pound loaves.

Basic Gluten-Free Bread

This is a nice, simple gluten-free recipe that can be a base for experimentation or a versatile sandwich standard. There might seem to be a lot of ingredients for such a basic bread, but after you make this once, the process will fall into place. You can throw nuts, raisins, and even fresh fruit into this bread for a nice variation.

- ¾ cup almond milk, at room temperature
- ½ cup garbanzo flour
- ¼ cup sorghum flour
- 2 tablespoons honey
- 1 tablespoon active dry yeast
- 1 teaspoon apple cider vinegar
- 2 large eggs, at room temperature
- 2 tablespoons extra-virgin olive oil
- ½ cup cornstarch
- ½ cup potato starch
- ½ cup tapioca flour
- 1 tablespoon xanthan gum
- 1 teaspoon sea salt
- Olive oil to grease loaf pan

1. In a medium bowl, whisk together the almond milk, garbanzo flour, sorghum flour, honey, yeast, and apple cider vinegar until well combined.

2. Cover the bowl and set in a warm place for 2–3 hours.

3. In a large bowl, beat the eggs well until foamy and then whisk in the oil.

4. Add the yeast mixture to the eggs and mix well.

5. In a small bowl, stir together the cornstarch, potato starch, tapioca flour, xanthan gum, and salt until well mixed.

6. Add the dry ingredients to the yeast mixture and beat to combine. You can add a little more almond milk if the dough seems too dry.

7. Beat the dough in a mixer on high speed for about 4 minutes.

8. Smooth the dough into a ball in the bowl and cover with plastic wrap.

9. Place the covered bowl in a warm spot to rise for about 35–45 minutes.

10. Preheat oven to 375 degrees F, and lightly grease an 8 x 4–inch loaf pan.

11. Transfer the dough to the loaf pan.

12. Bake for 55–60 minutes, until a knife inserted into the center comes out clean.

13. Allow the loaf to cool completely on a wire rack before removing it from the pan.

Makes 1 medium loaf.

Buckwheat Brown Bread

Buckwheat sounds like something you should not eat on a gluten-free diet. However, it is a fruit seed that is related to rhubarb, so it works quite well for people with gluten sensitivities. Eating foods that contain this versatile ingredient can also lower the risk of developing high blood pressure, high cholesterol, and certain cancers.

- 1½ cups gluten-free, all-purpose flour
- ½ cup buckwheat flour
- 2 tablespoons gluten-free baking powder
- 3 tablespoons granulated sugar
- ½ teaspoon sea salt
- 2 large egg whites
- 1 cup almond milk
- ½ cup extra-virgin olive oil, plus extra to grease loaf pan
- 2 tablespoons sesame seeds
- 1 tablespoon pine nuts

1. Preheat oven to 350 degrees F and lightly grease an 8 x 4–inch loaf pan.

2. In a large bowl, whisk together the flours, baking powder, sugar, and salt until well combined.

3. In a medium bowl, beat the egg whites until foamy. Add the almond milk and oil to the egg whites and stir to combine.

4. Add the wet ingredients to the dry and beat until the batter is smooth.

5. Spoon the batter into the loaf pan and smooth the top.

6. Sprinkle the top with the seeds and pine nuts, and bake for about 1 hour, until a knife inserted in the center comes out clean.

7. Let the loaf cool for 10 minutes. Then turn it out onto a wire rack until completely cool.

Makes 1 standard loaf (8–10 slices).

Seeded Honey Bread

Chia seeds are a lovely addition to many recipes that are part of health-oriented eating plans such as gluten-free, Paleo, raw, and vegan. These tiny seeds are over 20 percent protein, a complete protein (all eight essential amino acids), a great source of fiber, and high in antioxidants. Chia seeds can be used as an egg replacement if you are also sensitive to eggs, because when chia seeds are added to water, they form a gel that provides structure and helps leaven the dough.

- ¼ cup boiling water
- 4 teaspoons chia seeds
- ¾ cup warm water (110–115 degrees F)
- 1 teaspoon sugar
- 2 tablespoons active dry yeast
- 1 cup quinoa flour
- 1 cup brown rice flour
- ½ cup almond flour
- ½ cup potato starch
- 2 tablespoons pumpkin seeds
- 2 tablespoons sesame seeds
- 1 teaspoon sea salt
- 2 large eggs
- 2 tablespoons honey
- Coconut oil to grease loaf pan

1. Lightly grease a 9 x 5–inch loaf pan and set aside.

2. In a small bowl, stir together the chia seeds and boiling water, and set aside.

3. In another small bowl, stir together the warm water and sugar and then sprinkle the yeast over it. Set aside for about 10–15 minutes, until the yeast is foamy. Then stir again.

4. In a large bowl, combine the quinoa flour, brown rice flour, almond flour, potato starch, seeds, and salt until well mixed.

5. Add the eggs, honey, chia mixture, and yeast mixture to the dry ingredients, and beat to combine well.

6. Transfer the dough to the loaf pan and cover loosely with plastic wrap. Let the dough rise about 1 hour, until doubled in size.

7. Preheat oven to 400 degrees F.

8. Bake the bread for 10 minutes and then reduce the heat to 350 degrees F. Bake for an additional 30 minutes, until the bread is golden and a knife inserted into the center comes out clean.

9. Let the loaf cool for 10 minutes. Then turn it out onto a wire rack until completely cool.

Makes 1 standard loaf (8–10 slices).

Almost Cornbread

Cornbread is a steamy, buttery treat that should be eaten piping hot from the oven. This recipe does not actually use cornmeal, but it still manages to mimic cornbread quite well in texture and taste. The addition of jalapeños completes the flavor with a touch of heat. Do not substitute red chili flakes for fresh jalapeños, because in this case it will simply not be the same .

- 4 large eggs, at room temperature
- 1 cup warm water
- 4 teaspoons apple cider vinegar
- ¼ teaspoon minced garlic
- ½ teaspoon minced jalapeño pepper
- ¼ cup melted coconut oil, plus extra to grease loaf pans
- ½ cup of coconut flour
- ¼ teaspoon sea salt
- ½ tablespoon ground caraway seeds
- ½ teaspoon baking soda

1. Preheat oven to 350 degrees F and lightly grease two 2½ x 4½–inch mini loaf pans.

2. In a large bowl, beat together the eggs, water, apple cider vinegar, garlic, jalapeño pepper, and coconut oil until well combined.

3. In a small bowl, stir together the coconut flour, salt, caraway seeds, and baking soda.

4. Add the dry ingredients to the wet ingredients, and stir until completely blended.

5. Spoon the batter into the loaf pans and bake for about 45 minutes, or until a knife inserted in the center comes out clean.

6. Let the loaves cool for 10 minutes. Then turn them out onto a wire rack until completely cool.

Makes 2 mini loaves (8–10 slices in total).

Apple Parsnip Bread

This is really a fall bread bursting with moist apple, earthy parsnip, and warm spices. Parsnips are very high in fiber and are sweet without being overly high in calories. The fiber in parsnips can help lower cholesterol and regulate blood sugar. Parsnips are also high in folic acid and potassium, which can help cut the risk of dementia, cardiovascular disease, and birth defects.

- 1½ cups sifted almond flour
- 1½ teaspoons baking soda
- ¼ teaspoon salt
- ½ teaspoon ground cinnamon
- ¼ teaspoon ground nutmeg
- ¼ teaspoon ground ginger
- 3 large eggs
- 3 tablespoons pure maple syrup
- 1 tablespoon melted coconut oil, plus extra to grease loaf pans
- 1 cup grated apple
- 1 cup finely grated parsnip
- Almond flour to dust loaf pans

1. Preheat oven to 350 degrees F and lightly grease two 2½ x 4½–inch mini loaf pans and dust with almond flour.

2. In a small bowl, stir together the dry ingredients.

3. In a large bowl, whisk together the eggs, maple syrup, and coconut oil for about 3 minutes.

4. Whisk the apple and parsnip into the wet ingredients until well blended.

5. Add the dry ingredients to the wet ingredients and stir until combined.

6. Spoon the batter evenly into loaf pans and smooth the tops.

7. Bake for 35 minutes, until a knife inserted in the center comes out clean.

8. Let the loaves cool for 10 minutes. Then turn them out onto a wire rack until completely cool.

Makes 2 mini loaves (8–10 slices in total).

Multigrain Bread

Multigrain breads seem to be made specifically to be topped with robust fillings such as slices of turkey breast and chunky tuna salad. This loaf is studded with seeds and has a nutty, dense texture. Sesame seeds play an important role in the flavor of this bread and add to its health benefits. Sesame can lower cholesterol, help prevent high blood pressure, and protect the liver from oxidative damage.

- 1½ cups almond flour
- ¾ cup arrowroot powder
- ¼ cup flaxseed meal
- ¼ teaspoon salt
- ½ teaspoon baking soda
- 4 large eggs
- 2 teaspoons honey
- 1 teaspoon apple cider vinegar
- 2 tablespoons sesame seeds
- ½ cup hulled raw sunflower seeds
- Coconut oil to grease loaf pan

1. Preheat oven to 350 degrees F and lightly grease a 9 x 5–inch loaf pan.

2. In a medium bowl, stir together the almond flour, arrowroot powder, flaxseed meal, salt, and baking soda.

3. In a large bowl, beat the eggs with a hand mixer or whisk until very thick and frothy, about 5 minutes.

4. Beat the honey and apple cider vinegar into the eggs.

5. Gently fold the dry ingredients into the egg mixture until thoroughly mixed.

6. Fold in the sesame seeds and sunflower seeds.

7. Spoon the batter into the loaf pan, and bake for 40–45 minutes, until a knife inserted in the center comes out clean.

8. Let the loaf cool for 10 minutes. Then turn it out onto a wire rack until ready to serve. Serve warm whenever possible!

Makes 1 standard loaf (8–10 slices).

Gluten-Free Egg Bread

Egg bread is a tradition in many cultures, and this version is tender with the subtle crunch of sesame seeds. This loaf is the perfect base for French toast or as a before bed snack topped with homemade jam. You might have to drape a piece of foil over the bread while it is baking if it starts to get a little too brown.

- 2½ cups almond meal
- ⅓ cup tapioca flour
- ¾ teaspoon baking soda
- ¼ teaspoon sea salt
- 7 large eggs, at room temperature, divided
- ⅓ cup coconut oil, plus extra to grease loaf pan
- ⅓ cup coconut milk
- 4 teaspoons pure maple syrup
- 1 tablespoon sesame seeds

---

1. Preheat oven to 325 degrees F and lightly grease an 8½ x 4½–inch loaf pan. Line the bottom with parchment paper and lightly grease the parchment.

2. In a large bowl, stir together the almond meal, tapioca flour, baking soda, and salt until well combined.

3. In a small bowl, whisk together the egg yolks, coconut oil, coconut milk, and maple syrup.

4. Stir the egg mixture into the dry ingredients until smooth.

5. In a medium bowl, whisk the egg whites until they form moist, firm peaks.

6. Stir about one-third of the beaten egg whites into the batter to lighten it.

7. Carefully fold the remaining whites into the batter, taking care not to over mix.

8. Spoon the batter into the loaf pan, smoothing the top, and sprinkle with sesame seeds.

9. Bake bread for 40–45 minutes, until a knife inserted in the center comes out clean.

10. Let the loaf cool for 10 minutes. Then turn it out onto a wire rack until completely cool.

Makes 1 medium loaf (7–9 slices).

Sweet Almond Bread

This loaf is a triple dose of healthy almonds with almond flour, almond butter, and sliced almonds for topping. Almonds are a very important addition to any diet because they can help reduce the risk of high cholesterol and cardiovascular disease.

- ¾ cup almond butter
- 6 large eggs
- 4 teaspoons pure maple syrup
- ¼ cup coconut oil, plus extra to grease loaf pan
- ¼ cup flaxseed meal
- ¼ cup almond flour
- 4 teaspoons coconut flour
- ½ teaspoon baking soda
- ½ teaspoon salt
- 2 tablespoons toasted sliced almonds

1. Preheat oven to 350 degrees F and generously grease an 8 x 4–inch loaf pan.

2. In a large bowl, blend together the almond butter, eggs, maple syrup, and coconut oil with a hand mixer or whisk until smooth.

3. In a small bowl, combine the flaxseed meal, almond flour, coconut flour, baking soda, and salt.

4. Add the dry ingredients to the wet ingredients and blend together.

5. Spoon the batter into the loaf pan, and bake for 35–40 minutes, until a knife inserted in the center comes out clean.

6. Allow the bread to cool for 15 minutes, and then run a knife around the edges to remove from the pan. Then turn it out onto a wire rack until ready to serve. Serve warm or cold.

Makes 1 small loaf (6–8 slices).

Chia Bread

Chia seeds have quite amazing properties that make them a nice addition to a healthy diet. These little seeds can actually hold up to 12 times their weight in water and are popular for people trying to lose weight, because this gelling action can keep a person feeling full for hours. Chia seeds are a great source of omega-3 fatty acids as well as fiber. They can be found online and in the health-food section of most grocery stores.

- 1½ cups almond flour
- ½ cup coconut flour
- ¼ cup ground chia seeds or chia meal
- ½ teaspoon baking soda
- ¼ teaspoon sea salt
- 5 large eggs
- 4 tablespoons coconut oil, plus extra to grease loaf pan
- 1 tablespoon apple cider vinegar

1. Preheat oven to 350 degrees F and lightly grease an 8 x 4–inch loaf pan.

2. In a large bowl, stir together the almond flour, coconut flour, chia seeds, baking soda, and salt until well combined.

3. In a small bowl, whisk together the eggs, coconut oil, and apple cider vinegar.

4. Add the wet ingredients to the dry ingredients, and stir until incorporated completely.

5. Spoon into the loaf pan and smooth the top.

6. Bake for 40–50 minutes, until a knife inserted in the center comes out clean.

7. Let the loaf cool for 10 minutes. Then turn it out onto a wire rack until completely cool.

Makes 1 small loaf (6–8 slices).

Quinoa Sandwich Bread

This recipe is extremely simple and can be whipped together in less than 15 minutes and popped in the oven. Quinoa is a very versatile ingredient that can be ground down further if you want a finer texture to the bread. Quinoa boasts an impressive list of anti-inflammatory phytonutrients that are unique to this seed. Quinoa is also a good source of heart-healthy fats such as monounsaturated fat in the form of oleic acid.

- 1 cup whole quinoa
- 2 large eggs
- ¼ cup coconut flour

- 1 tablespoon melted coconut oil, plus extra to grease loaf pan
- 1 tablespoon water
- 1 tablespoon raw honey

1. Preheat the oven to 350 degrees F and lightly grease a 9 x 5–inch loaf pan.

2. Place the quinoa in a powerful blender, food processor, or clean coffee grinder, and process until it becomes a fine flour. Alternately, substitute with preground quinoa flour.

3. In a medium bowl, using an electric mixer, beat the eggs until light yellow and frothy.

4. In a large bowl, stir together the quinoa, coconut flour, and coconut oil until well combined. Stir in the water.

5. Add the eggs and honey to the flour mixture and stir until well combined.

6. Allow the dough to rest for 5 minutes, then stir again, adding a little more water if necessary to make the dough pliable and easy to knead. The dough should be lightly sticky, but not wet. Allow the dough to rest for 5 more minutes.

7. Place the dough in the loaf pan and bake for 30–35 minutes, until the top of the bread is golden brown and a knife inserted in the center comes out clean.

8. Allow the bread to cool completely on a wire rack before removing it from the pan.

Makes 1 standard loaf (8–10 slices).

Flax Bread with Fresh Herbs

Fresh herbs impart a lovely aroma to the whole house while this bread is baking. The herbs in this recipe have many health benefits such as helping improve digestion, stimulate the immune system, and increase circulation. The scent of rosemary has been shown to improve concentration because it increases blood flow to the brain. So try this fragrant loaf as a snack the next time important projects require your full attention.

- 1½ cups almond flour
- 3 tablespoons flaxseed meal
- 2 tablespoons coconut flour
- 1 tablespoon chopped fresh rosemary
- 1 teaspoon chopped fresh thyme
- 1 teaspoon chopped fresh oregano
- 1½ teaspoons baking soda
- ¼ teaspoon sea salt
- 5 large eggs
- ¼ cup coconut oil, plus extra to grease loaf pan
- 1 tablespoon apple cider vinegar

1. Preheat oven to 350 degrees F and lightly grease a 9 x 5–inch loaf pan.

2. In a large bowl, stir together the almond flour, flaxseed meal, coconut flour, herbs, baking soda, and salt until very well mixed.

3. In a medium bowl, whisk together the eggs, coconut oil, and apple cider vinegar.

4. Add the wet ingredients to the dry ingredients and stir to combine.

5. Spoon the batter into the loaf pan, and bake for 30–35 minutes, until a knife inserted in center comes out clean.

6. Let the loaf cool for 10 minutes. Then turn it out onto a wire rack until completely cool.

Makes 1 standard loaf (8–10 slices).

Black Olive Bread

This rustic Old World–style bread is infused with strong flavors and a satisfying dense texture. The cashew butter is rich and adds a smooth, almost buttery, component to the bread. Cashews are often placed in the nut category, but they are actually found on the bottom of the cashew apple and are classed as seeds. They are heart healthy and great for strong bones and teeth.

- ¼ cup almond flour
- ¼ cup arrowroot powder
- 1 teaspoon baking soda
- 3 large eggs
- ¾ cup natural raw cashew butter
- ½ cup pitted and chopped kalamata olives
- 1 tablespoon extra-virgin olive oil, plus extra to grease loaf pan

1. Preheat oven to 350 degrees F and lightly grease a 9 x 5–inch loaf pan.

2. In a medium bowl, stir together the almond flour, arrowroot powder, and baking soda until well combined.

3. In a large bowl, using an electric mixer, beat the eggs and cashew butter until well combined.

4. Add the flour mixture to the wet ingredients and stir until a wet dough forms.

5. Fold in the olives.

6. Spread the batter into the loaf pan and drizzle the olive oil over the top.

7. Bake for 25–30 minutes, until the top of the bread is golden brown.

8. Let the loaf cool for 10 minutes. Then turn it out onto a wire rack until completely cool.

Makes 1 standard loaf (8–10 slices).

Rhubarb Oat Bread

This pretty loaf might seem like it would be sweet, but the addition of rhubarb creates a tart flavor that complements meat and cheese sandwich fillings. Rhubarb is actually a vegetable but is usually treated similar to fruit in most recipes. Only the celery-like stalks are edible. The leaves contain oxalic acid and thus cannot be eaten—although fresh (not wilted) leaves are a great indicator of good rhubarb.

- 1 cup gluten-free rolled oats
- 1¼ cups boiling water
- ⅔ cup almond milk
- Juice of 1 lemon
- 1 cup buckwheat flour
- ½ cup gluten-free oat flour
- ½ cup tapioca flour
- ¾ cup granulated sugar
- ¼ cup ground chia seeds or chia meal
- 1 teaspoon baking soda
- 1 teaspoon gluten-free baking powder
- ½ teaspoon sea salt
- ⅓ cup melted coconut oil, plus extra to grease loaf pan
- 1 tablespoon pure vanilla extract
- 1 cup finely chopped fresh rhubarb

1. Preheat oven to 375 degrees F and lightly grease a 9 x 5–inch loaf pan.

2. Place the oats in a small bowl and pour the boiling water over them. Let sit for 2–4 minutes, stirring once, and then add the almond milk and lemon juice.

3. Let the oat mixture sit about 10 minutes until the oats are very soft.

4. In a large bowl, stir together the flours, sugar, ground chia seeds, baking soda, baking powder, and salt until well combined.

5. Add the oat mixture, coconut oil, and vanilla to the dry ingredients and stir to mix well.

6. Put the batter aside for a few minutes. Then add the chopped rhubarb.

7. Spoon the batter into the loaf pan and smooth the top.

8. Bake for 45–55 minutes, until a knife inserted in the center comes out clean.

9. Let the loaf cool for 10 minutes. Then turn it out onto a wire rack until completely cool.

Makes 1 standard loaf (8–10 slices).

Sun-Dried Tomato Bread

Sun-dried tomatoes are like concentrated sunshine and summer in neat, tender packages. They are sweet and lightly salty with a satisfying chewy texture. Make sure you get sun-dried tomatoes that are not like shoe leather but are rather those packed in flavorful oil or even dried in your own oven with a little olive oil and fresh cracked pepper. You can put more sun-dried tomatoes in this recipe if you want a more intense flavor.

- 1¼ cups warm water (110–115 degrees F)
- 1 teaspoon granulated sugar
- 1 packet active dry yeast
- 2 cups sorghum flour
- 1½ cups tapioca starch
- ½ cup gluten-free millet flour
- 2 tablespoons dried basil
- 1 tablespoon xanthan gum
- 1 teaspoon sea salt
- 1 tablespoon minced garlic, to taste
- 2 large eggs, beaten
- 3 tablespoons extra-virgin olive oil
- 1 teaspoon fresh lemon juice
- ¾ cup chopped sun-dried tomatoes

1. In a medium bowl, stir together the warm water and the sugar, and then sprinkle the yeast over the water. Set aside until the yeast gets foamy, about 10 minutes.

2. In a large bowl, mix together the sorghum flour, tapioca starch, millet flour, dried basil, xanthan gum, sea salt, and garlic until well combined.

3. Add the yeast mixture to the dry ingredients and beat to combine. Add the eggs, oil, and lemon juice to the dough, and beat until it is smooth. Add the sun-dried tomatoes into the dough and mix to incorporate.

4. Transfer the dough to a parchment-lined, 9-inch cake pan and smooth the top.

5. Place the pan in a warm spot and allow the dough to rise until about double in height, about an hour.

6. Preheat oven to 375 degrees F.

7. Bake for 30–35 minutes until golden and a knife inserted in the center comes out clean.

8. Let the loaf cool for 10 minutes. Then turn it out onto a wire rack until completely cool.

Makes 1 loaf (8–10 slices).

Pumpernickel Bread

If you are making a tasty spinach- or artichoke-cheese dip, and need a hearty, dense bread to accompany it, this is the perfect choice. This bread has a satisfying rustic crust and the deep, dark color of traditional pumpernickel. The color actually comes from the addition of cocoa, which has significant antioxidant and anti-inflammatory properties and can have a positive effect on mood.

- 1½ cups warm water (105–115 degrees F), divided
- 2 tablespoons active dry yeast
- 1 tablespoon granulated sugar
- 2 large eggs
- 2 large egg whites
- ¼ cup melted coconut oil, plus extra to grease dish
- ¼ cup apple cider vinegar
- ¼ cup dark molasses
- ¼ cup unsweetened apple juice
- 2 cups tapioca starch
- 1 cup buckwheat flour
- 1 cup flaxseed meal
- ½ cup cornstarch
- ¼ cup rice flour
- 4 tablespoons cocoa powder
- 2 tablespoons xanthan gum
- 1 teaspoon sea salt
- 1 tablespoon caraway seeds

1. Grease a large, round 2-quart casserole dish.

2. Place ½ cup of warm water in a medium bowl, and stir in the yeast and sugar. Let sit for about 10 minutes, until the yeast is foamy.

3. In a large bowl, stir together the remaining 1 cup of water, eggs, egg whites, coconut oil, apple cider vinegar, molasses, and apple juice until well blended.

4. In another medium bowl, mix together the tapioca starch, buckwheat flour, flaxseed meal, cornstarch, rice flour, cocoa powder, xanthan gum, and salt until combined.

5. Add the yeast mixture to the wet ingredients along with the dry ingredients and stir to combine. Beat the dough for about 4 minutes.

6. Transfer the dough to the casserole dish and sprinkle with the caraway seeds. Cover with plastic wrap. Let it sit in a warm spot until the dough rises above the rim of the dish, about 1 hour.

7. Preheat oven to 375 degrees F.

8. Bake for about 1 hour, covering the bread loosely with foil after 20 minutes to avoid over browning.

9. Let the loaf cool for 10 minutes. Then turn it out onto a wire rack until completely cool.

Makes 1 large loaf (12–15 slices).

Honey Flaxseed Sandwich Bread

Honey is a great way to add sweetness to bread without taking away from the other ingredients in the recipe. Honey contains a great deal of friendly bacteria, which may help control blood sugar and reduce the chance of insulin sensitivity. Honey also has been shown to boost immunity and improve metabolism issues.

- 1 cup almond flour
- ½ cup flaxseed meal
- 1 teaspoon baking soda
- 1 teaspoon cream of tartar
- 3 large eggs
- 2 tablespoons coconut oil, plus extra to grease loaf pan
- 2 tablespoons water
- 2 tablespoons raw honey

1. Preheat oven to 350 degrees F and lightly grease a 9 x 5–inch loaf pan.

2. In a medium bowl, stir together the flour, flaxseed meal, baking soda, and cream of tartar until well combined.

3. In a large bowl, using an electric mixer, beat the eggs until frothy. Add the coconut oil, water, and honey, and stir until well combined.

4. Add the flour mixture to the wet ingredients, and stir until incorporated.

5. Pour the batter into the loaf pan and bake for 25–30 minutes, until the top of the bread is dark brown and a knife inserted in the center comes out clean.

6. Allow the bread to cool completely on a wire rack before removing it from the pan.

Makes 1 standard loaf (8 to 10 slices).

Whole-Grain Olive Bread

If you like focaccia, you will also like this lovely golden bread. It is actually a flat loaf when finished, but the olives and herbs create a robust, satisfyingly salty taste. The loaf is surprisingly tender for such a rustic-looking creation, and you might be tempted to eat the whole thing in one sitting.

- 1 cup sorghum flour
- 1 cup quinoa flour
- ½ cup almond flour
- ¼ cup rice bran
- 2½ teaspoons active dry yeast
- 1 teaspoon xanthan gum
- 1 teaspoon garlic powder
- ½ teaspoon sea salt
- 3 large eggs, beaten
- ⅓ cup extra-virgin olive oil, plus extra to brush bread
- 1 tablespoon honey
- ½ cup warm water, or more if needed
- ½ cup pitted, sliced green olives
- Chopped fresh thyme, to taste

1. Preheat oven to 375 degrees F, and place a piece of parchment paper in a 9 x 12–inch baking sheet.

2. In a large bowl, stir together the sorghum flour, quinoa flour, almond flour, rice bran, yeast, xanthan gum, garlic powder, and sea salt until well combined.

3. In a small bowl, beat together the eggs, oil, and honey.

4. Make a well in the center of the dry ingredients and pour in the wet ingredients with the warm water. Stir to combine until the batter is smooth and a bit sticky. Add more water if needed.

5. Transfer the dough to the baking sheet and use your hands to form an oval loaf.

6. Stick the olive pieces all over the loaf, and then sprinkle the surface with thyme and salt.

7. Bake for 25 minutes, and then take it out and brush lightly with oil. Continue baking for another 10 minutes until bread is crusty and golden.

8. Allow the bread to cool on a wire rack for at least 15 minutes.

Makes 1 large loaf (12–14 slices).

Soft Sandwich Bread

This loaf has a surprise ingredient that helps create the tender, almost airy texture of this bread. Seltzer water can help create a nice rise in bread because it contains carbon dioxide bubbles, which create air pockets that expand in the heat of the oven. This bread is a lovely, light creation that is great for kids' sandwiches.

- 1¼ cups sorghum flour
- 1 cup brown rice flour, plus extra to dust loaf pan
- 1 cup potato starch
- ⅔ cup whey powder
- 2 tablespoons granulated sugar
- 1 packet instant yeast
- 3 teaspoons xanthan gum
- 1 teaspoon sea salt
- 2 large eggs, at room temperature
- ¼ cup melted coconut oil, plus extra to grease loaf pan
- 1¼ cups seltzer water, at room temperature

1. Preheat oven to 350 degrees F and lightly grease a 9 x 5–inch loaf pan. Then dust with brown rice flour.

2. In a large bowl, whisk together the sorghum flour, brown rice flour, potato starch, whey powder, sugar, yeast, xanthan gum, and salt.

3. In a small bowl, blend together the eggs and oil.

4. Add the egg mixture to the dry ingredients and slowly beat it in along with the seltzer water until a stretchy dough forms. Beat for about 4 minutes.

5. Transfer the dough to the loaf pan and smooth out the top. Cover the dough loosely with plastic wrap, and set in a warm spot until it rises above the rim of the pan, about 1 hour.

6. Using a serrated knife, score the top of the loaf three times, and bake for about 1 hour, until golden and a knife inserted in the

center comes out clean. While bread is baking, place a heavy cookie sheet in the oven along with the bread.

7. Remove the loaf from the pan and place it on the preheated cookie sheet. Bake for an additional 10–15 minutes or until the bread sounds hollow when tapped with the fingertips.

8. Let the loaf cool completely before slicing.

Makes 1 standard loaf (8–10 slices).

Basic Whole-Grain Bread

This recipe uses many different types of flours to create a tender, fragrant bread bursting with satisfying texture and taste. Oats are a nice addition, both for taste and the health benefits. Oats contain all the major nutrient groups needed by the body. They also digest very slowly, which keeps blood sugar stable.

- ½ cup warm water plus ⅓ cup (110–115 degrees F), divided
- 1 tablespoon honey
- 2½ teaspoons instant yeast
- ¾ cup sorghum flour
- ¾ cup almond flour
- ½ cup gluten-free oat flour
- ½ cup buckwheat flour
- 2 tablespoons coconut flour
- 1 teaspoon xanthan gum
- 1 teaspoon sea salt
- ¼ cup melted coconut oil
- 3 large eggs, beaten
- ¼ cup gluten-free oatmeal flakes

1. Place a piece of parchment paper in a 9 x 5–inch loaf pan.

2. Pour ½ cup of warm water in a small bowl and stir in the honey. Sprinkle the yeast on top and let stand for about 10 minutes, until it gets foamy.

3. In a large bowl, stir together the sorghum flour, almond flour, oat flour, buckwheat flour, coconut flour, xanthan gum, and sea salt until well combined.

4. Make a well in the center of the dry ingredients and add the yeast mixture along with the coconut oil and eggs.

5. Constantly beat the dough while adding the ⅓ cup of warm water, 1 tablespoon at a time. The batter should become smooth and thick, like muffin batter. Add more water if needed.

6. Transfer the bread dough to the loaf pan and smooth out the top. Sprinkle with oatmeal flakes. Let the dough rise for about an hour.

7. Preheat oven to 350 degrees F.

8. Bake for 55–60 minutes, until the loaf is crusty and browned and a knife inserted in the center comes out clean.

9. Let the loaf cool for 10 minutes. Then turn it out onto a wire rack until completely cool.

Makes 1 standard loaf (8–10 slices).

Brown Molasses Bread

This bread is brown because of the addition of molasses, which is full of healthy minerals and is a sweetener that can actually be considered good for you. Molasses is a very good source of iron, calcium, copper, manganese, potassium, and magnesium. It imparts a deep, almost bittersweet taste to this dense bread. This recipe also calls for grain teff, a staple of traditional Ethiopian cooking that adds a mild, nutty flavor.

- 2½ cups gluten-free, all-purpose flour
- ½ cup oat flour
- ¼ cup whole-grain teff
- 2 tablespoons granulated sugar
- 3 teaspoons instant yeast
- 2 teaspoons sea salt
- 1 teaspoon xanthan gum
- ¼ teaspoon baking soda
- 1 teaspoon apple cider vinegar
- ¼ teaspoon cream of tartar
- 2 extra-large egg whites, beaten
- 1½ cups warm milk (110–115 degrees F)
- ¼ cup unsalted butter, at room temperature, plus extra to grease loaf pan
- 1 tablespoon shortening, at room temperature
- 1 tablespoon unsulphured molasses

1. Lightly grease a 9 x 5–inch loaf pan.

2. In a large bowl, stir together the all-purpose flour, oat flour, teff, sugar, yeast, sea salt, xanthan gum, baking soda, and cream of tartar until well combined.

3. Add the egg whites, warm milk, butter, shortening, molasses, and vinegar. Mix until the dough comes together, and then, in an electric mixer, beat on high for about 5 minutes. The dough will be thick.

4. Scoop the dough into the loaf pan and cover loosely with plastic wrap. Place the pan in a warm spot and let it rise to just under double the volume.

5. Preheat oven to 375 degrees F.

6. Bake the bread for about 30 minutes, until it is firm, and then transfer it to a cookie sheet.

7. Place the loaf back in the oven, and bake for at least 10 more minutes, until it is hollow-sounding and golden and a knife inserted in the center comes out clean.

8. Allow the bread to cool on the cookie sheet for about 10 minutes, and then transfer it to a wire rack until completely cool.

Makes 1 standard loaf (8–10 slices).

Thyme Beer Bread

Beer is a very common ingredient in bread making because bread and beer share a common element: yeast. It is important to choose a gluten-free beer; however, also make sure you pick a beer that does not have a high alcohol content. Dark beer adds a richness to the bread that is enhanced when you toast the slices.

- 2½ cups gluten-free, all-purpose flour
- ⅓ cup whey powder
- ¼ cup light brown sugar
- 1½ teaspoons sea salt
- 1¼ teaspoons xanthan gum
- 1 teaspoon gluten-free baking powder
- ¼ teaspoon baking soda
- ¼ teaspoon cream of tartar
- 2 extra-large egg whites, at room temperature
- ¼ cup unsalted butter, at room temperature, plus extra to grease loaf pan and rub on bread
- ¾ cup gluten-free beer
- 1 tablespoon apple cider vinegar
- 3 tablespoons chopped fresh thyme

1. Preheat oven to 375 degrees F and lightly grease a 9 x 5–inch loaf pan.

2. In a large bowl, stir together the flour, whey powder, sugar, salt, xanthan gum, baking powder, baking soda, and cream of tartar until well combined.

3. Add the egg whites, butter, beer, and apple cider vinegar to the dry ingredients, and stir to combine. Beat until a soft dough forms. Add the thyme and mix to combine well.

4. Transfer the dough into the loaf pan and smooth the top.

5. Place a piece of aluminum foil, tented, over the loaf pan, and place the pan in the center of the oven.

6. Bake for 25 minutes. Then remove the foil and cut a slice lengthwise down the center of the bread.

7. Rub a little butter over the bread, and return it to the oven for another 20 minutes, until the loaf is golden and a knife inserted in the center comes out clean.

8. Let the loaf cool for 10 minutes. Then turn it out onto a wire rack until completely cool.

Makes 1 standard loaf (8–10 slices).

French-Style Baguettes

These loaves are crusty and golden with a hint of chewiness. Once you master this recipe, you will use this bread for sandwiches, dipping in soups, garlic bread, and perfect crostini for snacks. This recipe is easier with a heavy-duty mixer, but it also can be made quite well with a little arm work and a sturdy wooden spoon.

• 3 cups gluten-free, high-protein, all-purpose flour	• ¾ teaspoon salt
• 2 tablespoons instant yeast	• 1¼ cups warm water
• 1 tablespoon xanthan gum	• 2 large eggs, at room temperature
• 1 tablespoon granulated sugar	• 3 tablespoons extra-virgin olive oil, plus extra
• 1 tablespoon cornmeal, plus extra for dusting loaves	• 1 teaspoon apple cider vinegar

1. Preheat oven to 375 degrees F, and cover a cookie sheet with foil.

2. In a large bowl, stir together flour, yeast, xanthan gum, sugar, cornmeal, and salt until well combined.

3. In a medium bowl, whisk together the water, eggs, oil, and vinegar.

4. Add the wet ingredients to the dry ingredients.

5. Beat the mixture until well blended. Then beat for at least 5 minutes more.

6. Divide the dough in half, and with lightly oiled hands, shape into two baguettes.

7. Lightly oil each loaf, sprinkle each with cornmeal, and place on the cookie sheet. Cover the loaves with lightly oiled plastic wrap, and place in a warm place to rise for about 30 minutes.

8. Spritz the dough with water and place in the oven.

9. Bake for 30 minutes or until a toothpick inserted in the center comes out clean. Serve warm.

Makes 2 baguettes.

Pumpkin Sunflower-Seed Bread

This is a great bread for a grilled vegetable sandwich accented with creamy, tart goat cheese and fresh basil. Pumpkin is high in fiber, beta-carotene, vitamins A and C, potassium, and zinc. Make sure you grate the pumpkin very fine so the flavor and color are evenly dispersed.

- 3 cups finely grated pumpkin
- 4 large eggs
- ¼ cup coconut oil, plus extra to grease loaf pan
- 2 tablespoons honey
- 1 tablespoon fresh lemon juice
- 3 cups almond flour
- ¾ teaspoon baking soda
- ½ teaspoon sea salt
- ½ teaspoon ground nutmeg
- 2 tablespoons hulled raw sunflower seeds

1. Preheat oven to 325 degrees F and lightly grease a 9 x 5–inch loaf pan. Line the bottom of the pan with parchment paper, and grease the parchment.

2. In a large bowl, stir together the pumpkin, eggs, coconut oil, honey, and lemon juice until well mixed.

3. In a small bowl, stir together the almond flour, baking soda, salt, and nutmeg.

4. Add the dry ingredients to the wet ingredients, and stir until well incorporated.

5. Spoon the batter into the loaf pan, and sprinkle the top with sunflower seeds.

6. Bake for about 1–1½ hours, until a knife inserted in the center comes out clean.

7. Let the loaf cool for 1 hour. Then turn it out onto a wire rack until completely cool.

Makes 1 standard loaf (8–10 slices).

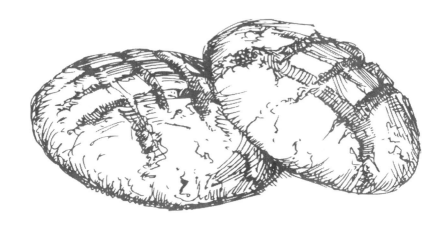

Without wishing in the slightest degree to disparage the skill and labour of breadmakers by trade, truth compels us to assert our conviction of the superior wholesomeness of bread made in our own homes.

—Eliza Acton

3

SWEET AND SUMPTUOUS BREADS

Coconut Yam Bread

This loaf is sweet, tender, and a pretty golden color. Yams provide the daily recommended serving of potassium and magnesium and are also a great source of all the B vitamins. If you add coconut to all that goodness, you have a nutrition-packed loaf that makes for a great breakfast toast. Coconut is linked to improved digestion, higher energy, and increased endurance.

- 2 cups all-purpose, gluten-free flour
- 1 cup shredded unsweetened coconut
- 1 tablespoon gluten-free baking powder
- 1 teaspoon ground cinnamon
- Pinch of sea salt
- 2 large eggs
- 1 cup coconut milk
- ¾ cup pureed baked yam
- ½ cup granulated sugar
- 4 tablespoons plain Greek yogurt
- 2 tablespoons melted coconut oil, plus extra to grease loaf pan
- 1 teaspoon pure vanilla extract

1. Preheat oven to 350 degrees F and generously grease a 9 x 5–inch loaf pan.

2. In a medium bowl, stir together the flour, coconut, baking powder, cinnamon, and salt until well combined.

3. In a large bowl, beat together the eggs, coconut milk, pureed yam, sugar, yogurt, coconut oil, and vanilla until well blended.

4. Add the dry ingredients to the wet ingredients and stir until just combined.

5. Spoon the batter into the loaf pan and smooth the top.

6. Bake for 60–65 minutes, until a knife inserted in the center comes out clean.

7. Let the loaf cool for 10 minutes. Then turn it out onto a wire rack until completely cool.

Makes 1 standard loaf (8–10 slices).

Chocolate Carrot Bread

Moist carrot, crunchy pecans, rich dark chocolate, and creamy thick Greek yogurt all combine to create an exceptional bread. Most natural yogurts are healthy, but Greek-style yogurt might be one of the best foods in the world to include in a nutritionally sound diet. This yogurt has probiotic cultures and twice the protein of regular yogurts, which also makes this bread very tender.

- 1½ cups almond flour
- 4 tablespoons cocoa powder
- 2 teaspoons ground cinnamon
- 1½ teaspoons baking soda
- Pinch of sea salt
- 1 large egg, at room temperature
- 4 tablespoons plain Greek yogurt
- 4 tablespoons melted coconut oil
- 3 tablespoons honey
- 1 teaspoon apple cider vinegar
- 1 teaspoon pure vanilla extract
- 1 cup finely grated carrot
- ¾ cup chopped pecans
- ½ cup gluten-free chocolate chips

1. Preheat oven to 350 degrees and line an 8½ x 4½–inch loaf pan with parchment paper.

2. In a medium bowl, stir together the almond flour, cocoa powder, cinnamon, baking soda, and salt until well mixed.

3. In a large bowl, whisk together the egg, yogurt, coconut oil, honey, apple cider vinegar, and vanilla until well blended. Stir in the grated carrot, pecans, and chocolate chips until incorporated.

4. Add the dry ingredients and stir until just combined.

5. Transfer the batter to the loaf pan and bake for 35–40 minutes, until a knife inserted in the center comes out clean.

6. Let the loaf cool for 10 minutes. Then turn it out onto a wire rack until completely cool.

Makes 1 medium loaf (6–8 slices).

Cinnamon Pear Bread

Pears are an underused ingredient in breads and other baking because people usually think of apples first. Pears are sweet, slightly grainy, and packed with nutrition. It is important to leave the skin on the pears in this recipe to produce the best results. Studies have shown that pear skins contain antioxidants, anti-inflammatory flavonoids, and close to half of the pear's total dietary fiber. Try to find pears that are just ripe rather than really soft, or it will be impossible to grate them.

- 1½ cups brown rice flour
- ½ cup tapioca flour
- 1 tablespoon ground cinnamon
- 1 teaspoon gluten-free baking powder
- 1 teaspoon sea salt
- 2 large eggs
- 1¼ cups granulated sugar
- ½ cup melted coconut oil, plus extra to grease loaf pan
- 1 tablespoon pure vanilla extract
- 2 large almost-ripe pears, cored and finely grated
- 1 cup chopped pecans
- Brown rice flour to dust loaf pan

---

1. Preheat oven to 350 degrees F. Lightly grease a 9 x 5–inch loaf pan and dust with brown rice flour.

2. In a large bowl, stir together the brown rice flour, tapioca flour, cinnamon, baking powder, and salt until well combined.

3. In a small bowl, whisk together the eggs, sugar, coconut oil, and vanilla until well blended.

4. Add the wet ingredients to the dry ingredients and stir until just combined.

5. Add the grated pear and pecans to the batter and stir to combine.

6. Spoon the batter into the loaf pan.

7. Bake for 60–65 minutes, until a knife inserted in the center comes out clean.

8. Let the loaf cool for 10 minutes. Then turn it out onto a wire rack until completely cool.

Makes 1 standard loaf (8–10 slices).

Apple Scones

Scones can be a truly spectacular addition to a leisurely Sunday morning or afternoon tea break. These scones are a tribute to apples and feature juicy chunks of fruit in apple butter. Apple butter is a great source of insoluble fiber and vitamins A and C. This is important for healthy digestion, teeth, and skin.

- 1 cup millet flour
- 1 cup sorghum flour
- ½ cup rice flour
- ½ cup potato starch
- 1 teaspoon gluten-free baking powder
- 1 teaspoon xanthan gum
- ½ teaspoon baking soda
- ½ teaspoon sea salt
- ⅔ cup apple butter
- ⅓ cup agave nectar
- ¼ cup palm oil shortening
- 1 cup peeled and diced tart apples

1. Preheat oven to 375 degrees F and cover a cookie sheet with parchment paper.

2. In a large bowl, mix together the flours, potato starch, baking powder, xanthan gum, baking soda, and salt until well combined.

3. With a fork, beat in the apple butter, agave, and shortening until just combined. Add the diced apples and mix to combine.

4. Pat the dough out into a circle and use a knife to cut it into eight equal pie-shaped pieces.

5. Place on the cookie sheet and bake for 15–20 minutes, until they are golden brown and a knife inserted in the center comes out clean.

6. Cool for about 15 minutes before serving.

Makes 8 scones.

Applesauce Spice Bread

This loaf is a simple, tasty, snack-style bread that is better served completely chilled. Applesauce is a great way to create moist, tender, textured bread without added calories or fat. You can also use mashed cooked apple if you don't have any store-bought product in your pantry. This recipe would also be very nice with pear instead of apple, especially if you toss in a dash of nutmeg, as well.

- 2 cups almond flour
- 1 tablespoon ground cinnamon
- 1 teaspoon baking soda
- 2 large eggs
- ½ cup cold water
- ¼ cup pure maple syrup
- 1 teaspoon pure vanilla extract
- ½ cup unsweetened applesauce
- 1 large apple, peeled, cored, and chopped
- ¼ cup chopped pecans
- Coconut oil to grease loaf pan

1. Preheat oven to 350 degrees F and lightly grease a 9 x 5–inch loaf pan.

2. In a medium bowl, sift together the almond flour, cinnamon, and baking soda until well combined.

3. In a large bowl, using an electric mixer, beat the eggs until frothy. Add the water, maple syrup, and vanilla, and stir until well combined. Stir in the applesauce, and then fold in the chopped apple.

4. Carefully add the flour mixture to the wet ingredients and stir until just combined.

5. Pour the batter into the loaf pan and sprinkle the pecans over the top.

6. Bake for 35–40 minutes, until the top of the bread is browned and the edges are crisp and a knife inserted into the center should come out clean.

7. Allow the bread to cool completely on a wire rack before removing it from the pan.

Makes 1 standard loaf (8–10 slices).

Pumpkin Honey Bread

If you can imagine crisp autumn evenings in bread form, this loaf would come quite close. It is a little like pumpkin pie but not as sweet. If you want a slightly different taste, you can also use mashed slow-roasted butternut squash with a little butter and brown sugar instead of pumpkin. If you use squash, you should also substitute maple syrup for honey because it is a better combination.

- 1 cup almond flour
- 1 teaspoon baking soda
- 2 teaspoons ground cinnamon
- ¼ teaspoon ground nutmeg
- ¼ teaspoon ground cloves
- ½ cup pumpkin puree (canned or freshly roasted)
- 3 tablespoons raw honey
- 3 large eggs
- Coconut oil to grease loaf pan

1. Preheat the oven to 350 degrees F and lightly grease a 9 x 5–inch loaf pan.

2. In a medium bowl, stir together the almond flour, baking soda, cinnamon, nutmeg, and cloves.

3. In a large bowl, using an electric mixer, beat the pumpkin puree, honey, and eggs until frothy.

4. Carefully add the flour mixture to the wet ingredients and stir until just combined.

5. Pour the batter into the loaf pan and bake for 30–40 minutes, until the top of the bread is lightly browned and a knife inserted in the center comes out clean.

6. Allow the bread to cool completely on a wire rack before removing it from the pan.

Makes 1 standard loaf (8–10 slices).

Lemon Poppy Seed Bread

This is a very classic combination. The poppy seeds provide a lovely little crunch to this tart bread while imparting some serious health benefits as well. Poppy seeds come from the glorious opium poppy, which is also the source of morphine. Poppy seeds contain calcium, iron, and zinc and are rich in oleic and linoleic acid. This means they are beneficial to almost every system in the body.

- 2 cups almond flour
- 2 teaspoons gluten-free baking powder
- 4 large eggs
- ½ cup coconut oil, plus extra to grease loaf pan
- 5 tablespoons raw honey
- Zest of 2 lemons
- ¼ cup water
- ¼ cup lemon juice
- 2 tablespoons poppy seeds

1. Preheat the oven to 350 degrees F and lightly grease a 9 x 5–inch loaf pan.

2. In a medium bowl, stir together the almond flour and baking powder until combined.

3. In a large bowl, using an electric mixer, beat the eggs, coconut oil, and honey. Add the zest, water, and juice and stir to combine.

4. Add the flour mixture to the wet ingredients and stir until well combined.

5. Fold in the poppy seeds.

6. Pour the batter into the loaf pan and bake for 30–40 minutes, or until a knife inserted in the center comes out clean.

7. Allow the bread to cool completely on a wire rack before removing it from the pan.

Makes 1 standard loaf (8–10 slices).

The Best Banana Bread

This should be a staple recipe in any kitchen, gluten-free or otherwise, because it tastes just as banana bread is meant to taste. You have to make sure your bananas are very ripe to get the right texture and sweetness in the bread. If you have too many ripe bananas, you can place them in the freezer for future use. Simply thaw them out and mash when you are ready to bake.

- 3 ripe bananas, mashed
- 3 large eggs
- ¼ cup honey
- 3 tablespoons coconut oil, plus extra to grease loaf pan
- 2 tablespoons coconut cream (the thick layer at the top of a can of coconut milk)
- 1½ cups almond flour
- 3 tablespoons tapioca flour
- 2 tablespoons shredded unsweetened coconut
- 1 teaspoon gluten-free baking powder
- 1 teaspoon ground cinnamon
- ½ cup chopped pecans

---

1. Preheat oven to 325 degrees F. Grease an 8½ x 4½–inch loaf pan and line the bottom with parchment paper. Grease the parchment as well.

2. In a large bowl, beat together with a hand mixer the banana, eggs, honey, coconut oil, and coconut cream until well mixed.

3. In a medium bowl, stir together the remaining ingredients (except the pecans) to combine.

4. Add the dry ingredients to the banana mixture and beat to incorporate.

5. Spoon the batter into the loaf pan and smooth the surface. Sprinkle the top with the pecans.

6. Bake for 45 minutes, until a knife inserted in the center comes out clean.

7. Let the loaf cool for 10 minutes. Then turn it out onto a wire rack until completely cool.

Makes 1 medium loaf (7-9 slices).

Cherry Pumpkin Bread

Dried cherries are used to great effect in this rich, tender crumb bread, creating a flavor that is tart, sweet, and intensely cherry. A little dried cherry goes a long way, so do not be tempted to add any more. These powerhouse morsels can help cut the risk of diabetes as well as cardiovascular disease, assist in weight loss, and help cut cholesterol. You could substitute dried cranberries in this recipe, but the results are not as sublime.

- 1 overripe banana, mashed
- ¼ cup canned pumpkin puree
- 2 tablespoons coconut oil, plus extra to grease loaf pan
- 2 large eggs
- 1 tablespoon raw honey
- 1 tablespoon pure vanilla extract
- 2 cups almond flour
- 1 teaspoon baking soda
- 1 teaspoon gluten-free baking powder
- ½ teaspoon ground cinnamon
- ½ cup unsweetened dried cherries
- ¼ cup 70 percent dark chocolate chips

1. Preheat oven to 350 degrees F and lightly grease a 9 x 5–inch loaf pan.

2. In a large bowl, combine the mashed banana, pumpkin puree, and oil. Add the eggs, one at a time, followed by the honey and vanilla, and stir well to combine.

3. In a medium bowl, combine the almond flour, baking soda, baking powder, and cinnamon.

4. Add the flour mixture to the wet ingredients and stir until well combined.

5. Carefully fold in the cherries and chocolate chips.

6. Pour the batter into the loaf pan and bake for 35–40 minutes, until the top of the bread is browned and a knife inserted in the center comes out clean.

7. Allow the bread to cool completely on a wire rack before removing it from the pan.

Makes 1 standard loaf (8–10 slices).

Orange Honey Bread

Simple can sometimes be better, especially in the case of this easy-to-prepare loaf. The flavor of this loaf is pure and clean with no spices to distract from the essence of orange. Make sure you wash your oranges well before removing the zest. This gets rid of any pesticides or other harmful elements on the skin.

- 3½ cups almond flour
- ½ teaspoon gluten-free baking powder
- 5 large eggs
- Juice of 2 large oranges, strained
- Zest of 1 orange
- ¼ cup honey
- 1 tablespoon apple cider vinegar
- 2 tablespoons sliced almonds
- Coconut oil to grease loaf pan

1. Preheat oven 350 degrees F and lightly grease a 9 x 5–inch loaf pan.

2. In a medium bowl, stir together the almond flour and baking powder.

3. In a large bowl, whisk the eggs, orange juice, zest, honey, and apple cider vinegar until well blended.

4. Add the dry ingredients to the wet ingredients and stir to combine.

5. Spoon the batter into the loaf pan and sprinkle with the almonds.

6. Bake for 40–45 minutes, until a knife inserted in the center comes out clean.

7. Let the loaf cool for 10 minutes. Then turn it out onto a wire rack until completely cool.

Makes 1 standard loaf (8–10 slices).

Chocolate Cherry Bread

This loaf will remind you of Black Forest cake because of the rich chocolate and fresh juicy cherries. It is best to pit the cherries ahead of time and let them sit in a strainer for a few hours so that the bread does not get too soggy. The cherries should be ripe for the best results, and if they are a little tart, toss them in some sugar first.

- ½ cup coconut flour
- ½ cup flaxseed meal
- 1 teaspoon baking soda
- 2 teaspoons ground cinnamon
- 1 teaspoon sea salt
- 6 large eggs
- 3 large bananas, mashed
- 1 tablespoon pure vanilla extract
- 1 cup pitted fresh cherries
- 2 tablespoons cocoa powder
- 2 teaspoons coconut milk
- Coconut oil to grease loaf pan

1. Preheat oven to 350 degrees F and lightly grease a 9 x 5–inch loaf pan.

2. In a medium bowl, stir together the coconut flour, flaxseed meal, baking soda, cinnamon, and salt until combined.

3. In a large bowl, beat together the eggs, bananas, and vanilla until well blended.

4. Add the dry ingredients in small amounts to the wet ingredients and stir to combine.

5. Spread the fresh cherries in the bottom of the loaf pan, and pour two-thirds of the batter over them.

6. Add the cocoa powder and coconut milk to the leftover batter, and stir to combine.

7. Spoon the chocolate batter over the other batter, and use a knife to swirl the chocolate batter through in a marble pattern.

8. Bake for about 50 minutes, until a knife inserted in the center comes out clean.

9. Allow the bread to cool completely on a wire rack before removing it from the pan. Serve cherry side up.

Makes 1 standard loaf (8–10 slices).

Cranberry Orange Bread

Cranberries add a gorgeous jewel-like appearance to this loaf, which is enhanced by the addition of sunny-hued orange zest. It seems almost Christmassy in nature, but the flavors are actually perfect for a hot summer day. Cranberries are wonderful for the immune system because they contain powerful antioxidants and vitamin C.

- ⅔ cup coconut flour
- 2 teaspoons gluten-free baking powder
- 1 teaspoon baking soda
- 1 teaspoon sea salt
- Juice of 2 large oranges
- Zest of ½ orange
- 2 medium-ripe bananas, mashed
- ¼ cup coconut oil, plus extra to grease loaf pan
- 4 large eggs, lightly beaten
- 3 tablespoons honey
- ½ cup dried cranberries, cut in half

1. Preheat oven to 350 degrees F and lightly grease a 9 x 5–inch loaf pan.

2. In a large bowl, stir together the coconut flour, baking powder, baking soda, and salt until very well combined.

3. In a medium bowl, whisk together the orange juice, zest, bananas, and coconut oil until blended. Add the eggs and stir to combine.

4. Add the wet ingredients to the dry ingredients and stir to combine.

5. Add the honey and cranberries to the batter, and stir to combine.

6. Spoon the batter into the loaf pan and smooth the top.

7. Bake for about 1 hour, until a knife inserted in the center comes out clean.

8. Let the loaf cool for 10 minutes. Then turn it out onto a wire rack until completely cool.

Makes 1 standard loaf (8–10 slices).

Cashew Date Bread

This bread is studded with rich pieces of cashew and sweet dates—an addictive combination! Dates are not a common ingredient in Western recipes except perhaps for cookies; however, they are very healthy and can help fight intestinal disorders and abdominal cancer. Dates are also a natural source of energy, which can be felt as little as half an hour after eating them.

- 1 cup almond flour
- 1 tablespoon ground cinnamon
- ½ teaspoon baking soda
- ¼ teaspoon sea salt
- 3 large eggs
- 2 tablespoons pure maple syrup
- 1 teaspoon pure vanilla extract
- ¾ cup chopped cashews
- ½ cup chopped dates
- Coconut oil to grease loaf pan

1. Preheat oven to 350 degrees F. Lightly grease a 9 x 5–inch loaf pan and line the bottom of the pan with parchment; set aside.

2. In a large bowl, stir together all the ingredients except the cashews and dates until well combined.

3. Gently stir in the cashews and dates.

4. Spoon batter into loaf pan.

5. Bake bread for 35 minutes, until a knife inserted in the center comes out clean.

6. Let the loaf cool in the pan for 15 minutes and then remove it from the pan.

7. Store this bread overnight before serving.

Makes 1 standard loaf (8–10 slices).

Zucchini Bread

Zucchini has an interesting, almost porous, texture that is very good for baking bread. Zucchini is a wonderful source of beta-carotene and is a mild diuretic, which means your bread will also be a healthy addition to your day. You can substitute with yellow squash with little effect on taste and appearance.

- 1½ cups almond flour
- 1 teaspoon baking soda
- 1 teaspoon ground cinnamon
- ½ teaspoon ground nutmeg
- Pinch of ground ginger
- ½ teaspoon sea salt
- 3 large eggs, lightly beaten
- ¼ cup honey
- 1 large ripe banana, mashed
- 1 cup shredded zucchini, squeezed lightly
- Coconut oil to grease loaf pans

1. Preheat oven to 350 degrees F and lightly grease two 2½ x 4½–inch mini loaf pans.

2. In a medium bowl, stir together the almond flour, baking soda, spices, and salt.

3. In a large bowl, whisk together the eggs, honey, banana, and zucchini for about 2 minutes until very well mixed.

4. Add the dry ingredients to the wet ingredients and stir to combine.

5. Spoon the bread batter into the loaf pans.

6. Bake bread for 30–35 minutes, until a knife inserted in the center comes out clean.

7. Let the loaf cool for 10 minutes. Then turn it out onto a wire rack until completely cool.

Makes 2 small loaves (8–10 slices).

Coconut Banana Bread

This loaf is infused with tropical tastes and scents that are pleasing to the palate and beneficial for the body. One of the well-known minerals in bananas is potassium, which is crucial for regulating blood pressure and helping prevent muscle cramps. Bananas also provide fiber, vitamin B6, vitamin C, and manganese in a neat, low-calorie package. This bread is a convenient way to get all this goodness at once.

- ¾ cup almond flour
- ¼ cup coconut flour
- ¾ teaspoon baking soda
- ¾ teaspoon gluten-free baking powder
- ½ teaspoon sea salt
- ¾ teaspoon ground cinnamon
- ¼ teaspoon ground ginger
- ¼ teaspoon ground nutmeg
- 2 large eggs
- ⅓ cup pure maple syrup
- 2 tablespoons melted coconut oil, plus extra to grease loaf pan
- 1 teaspoon pure vanilla extract
- 2 large very ripe bananas, mashed
- ¼ cup shredded unsweetened coconut
- Almond flour to dust the loaf pan

1. Preheat oven to 350 degrees F. Lightly grease a 9 x 5–inch loaf pan and dust it with almond flour.

2. In a large bowl, sift together the flours, baking soda, baking powder, salt, and spices.

3. In a small bowl, whisk together the eggs, maple syrup, coconut oil, and vanilla until well combined. Whisk in the bananas and shredded coconut.

4. Add the wet ingredients to the dry ingredients and stir together until just combined. Do not overmix the batter or the bread will be too dense.

5. Spoon the batter into the loaf pan.

6. Bake for about 55 minutes, until a knife inserted in the center comes out clean.

7. Let the loaf cool for 20 minutes. Then turn it out onto a wire rack until completely cool.

Makes 1 standard loaf (8–10 slices).

Double Lemon Bread

This bread is tart, sweet, and decadent. It has a very strong lemon taste that is enhanced by the glaze. Lemon is one of the most popular flavors for baking, and it is also very healthy. It is high in vitamin C, which makes it a very effective treatment for infections and to detoxify the body. Lemons are also used to treat many digestive issues such as nausea and heartburn.

For the bread:

- 6 large eggs
- 4 tablespoons coconut oil, plus extra to grease loaf pan
- Juice from 2 lemons
- ⅔ cup coconut milk or enough to make 1 cup liquid when added to the lemon juice
- Zest from 2 lemons
- ½ cup honey
- ⅔ cup coconut flour
- 1½ teaspoons baking soda
- ¼ teaspoon sea salt

For the glaze:

- Zest and juice from 1 large lemon
- 2 tablespoons coconut milk
- 4 teaspoons coconut oil
- 3 teaspoons honey, or to taste
- ½ teaspoon pure vanilla extract

Make the bread:

1. Preheat oven to 350 degrees F and lightly grease an 8 x 4–inch loaf pan.

2. In a large bowl, whisk together the eggs, coconut oil, lemon juice, coconut milk, lemon zest, and honey until incorporated.

3. In a small bowl, stir together the coconut flour, baking soda, and salt.

4. Add the dry ingredients to the wet ingredients and stir to combine well.

5. Spoon the batter into the loaf pan.

6. Bake for 35–45 minutes, until golden brown and a knife inserted in the center comes out clean.

7. Let cool for 10 minutes and then remove from the pan. Then turn it out onto a wire rack until ready to glaze.

Make the glaze:

8. When the lemon loaf comes out of the oven, combine all the ingredients for the glaze in a small saucepan over low heat.

9. Stir constantly until the glaze comes to a simmer, and then remove from the heat.

10. Cool for at least 15 minutes. Place a piece of foil or parchment paper under the wire rack, and then slowly pour the glaze over the lemon bread.

11. Place the bread in the refrigerator for at least 1 hour until the glaze firms up.

Makes 1 small loaf (6-8 slices).

Apple Cream-Cheese Bread

This bread has layers of tender apple, creamy cheesecake, and a sweet almond-scented glaze. And the trick to its melt-in-your-mouth texture is to fold the egg whites very carefully into the batter—keeping as much volume as possible. This is a great bread to bring as a hostess gift or as a housewarming present.

For the filling:
- 8 ounces cream cheese
- ½ cup granulated sugar
- 1 large egg
- 2 teaspoons gluten-free, all-purpose flour
- 1 teaspoon pure vanilla extract

For the glaze:
- 4 teaspoons granulated sugar
- 1–2 teaspoons almond milk
- ½ teaspoon pure vanilla extract

For the bread:
- ½ cup unsalted butter, plus extra to grease the loaf pan
- ½ cup brown sugar
- 1 teaspoon pure vanilla extract
- Pinch of sea salt
- 2 large eggs, separated
- 1½ cups gluten-free, all-purpose flour, plus extra to dust the pan
- 1 teaspoon gluten-free baking powder
- ⅓ cup almond milk
- 2 cups diced apple
- 3 tablespoons granulated sugar

Make the filling:
1. In a medium bowl, beat together the cream cheese and sugar until very smooth. Add the egg and beat until incorporated, scraping down the sides of the bowl.

2. Add the flour and vanilla, and beat until smooth. Set aside.

Make the glaze:

3. In a small bowl stir together all the ingredients and set aside.

Make the bread:

4. Preheat oven to 350 degrees F. Lightly grease a 9 x 5–inch loaf pan and dust it with gluten-free flour.

5. In a large bowl, beat together the butter and brown sugar until well combined and fluffy. Add the vanilla and salt, and beat again. Add the egg yolks and beat to combine, scraping down the sides of the bowl.

6. In a medium bowl, stir together the flour and baking powder until well mixed.

7. Add the flour mixture and almond milk to the butter mixture in three alternating steps—starting and finishing with the flour. Add the apple to the batter.

8. In a separate large bowl, beat the egg whites until soft peaks form. Then add the sugar, 1 tablespoon at a time, until stiff peaks form.

9. Carefully fold the egg whites into the batter.

10. Spoon half of the bread batter into the loaf pan and spoon the filling over the layer of batter. Spoon the remaining batter over the filling. Spoon the glaze over the top of the bread.

11. Bake for 50–60 minutes, until a knife inserted in the center comes out clean.

12. Let the loaf cool for 20 minutes. Then turn it out onto a wire rack until completely cool. Serve chilled.

Makes 1 standard loaf (8–10 slices).

Chocolate Gingerbread Bread

Gingerbread is a comfort food that is made even better with the addition of chocolate. Ginger has been used for centuries to treat health issues and flavor culinary creations, and it has many medicinal applications and benefits. It is effective for digestive system complaints such as nausea or indigestion and can also be a powerful anti-inflammatory, which can treat arthritis and help fight free radicals in the body.

- 1 cup sorghum flour
- 1 cup light brown sugar
- ¾ cup almond flour
- ½ cup potato starch
- ⅓ cup cocoa powder
- 2 teaspoons gluten-free baking powder
- 2 teaspoons ground ginger
- 1 teaspoon ground cinnamon
- 1 teaspoon xanthan gum
- ¾ teaspoon baking soda
- ¾ teaspoon sea salt
- ½ teaspoon ground nutmeg
- 2 large eggs, lightly beaten
- ½ cup unsulphured molasses
- ¼ cup almond milk
- ¼ cup melted coconut oil
- 2 teaspoons pure vanilla extract

1. Preheat oven to 350 degrees F. Line a 9 x 5–inch loaf pan with parchment paper all the way up the sides of the pan.

2. In a large bowl, stir together the sorghum flour, brown sugar, almond flour, potato starch, cocoa powder, baking powder, ginger, cinnamon, xanthan gum, baking soda, sea salt, and nutmeg until well combined.

3. Make a well in the center, and add the eggs, molasses, almond milk, coconut oil, and vanilla. Mix until the batter is smooth.

4. Transfer the batter to the loaf pan and bake for 50–60 minutes, until a knife inserted in the center comes out clean.

5. Let the loaf cool for about 30 minutes before turning it out onto a wire rack to cool completely before serving.

Makes 1 standard loaf (8–10 slices).

Lemon-Scented Soda Bread

Soda bread is a traditional bread that uses baking soda instead of yeast as a leavening agent. This version is flavored with tart lemon and fresh orange juice. The oat and rice flour in this recipe combine nicely to create a tender crumb in the loaf.

- 1 cup gluten-free oat flour
- 1 cup potato starch
- ½ cup sorghum flour
- ¾ cup packed light brown sugar
- 2 teaspoons xanthan gum
- 1½ teaspoons gluten-free baking powder
- 1 teaspoon baking soda
- ¾ teaspoon sea salt
- ⅓ cup coconut oil
- ½ cup freshly squeezed orange juice
- ¼ cup fresh lemon juice
- 2 large eggs, beaten
- 1 tablespoon lemon zest

1. Preheat the oven to 350 degrees F. Line the bottom of an 8-inch round cake pan with parchment paper.

2. In a large bowl, mix together the oat flour, potato starch, sorghum flour, light brown sugar, xanthan gum, baking powder, baking soda, and sea salt until well combined.

3. Using your fingers, rub in the coconut oil (which should be solid) until the mixture resembles crumbs.

4. Add in the orange juice, lemon juice, eggs, and lemon zest. Stir until a smooth dough forms.

5. Transfer the dough to the cake pan and form into a round loaf. Smooth down the top and make an "X" on top with a knife.

6. Bake for 30–35 minutes, until the loaf is firm and slightly golden.

7. Let the loaf cool for 10 minutes. Then turn it out onto a wire rack until completely cool.

Makes one round loaf (8–10 slices).

Cinnamon-Scented Banana Bread

The scent of cinnamon often brings people back to wonderful memories because it is present in many traditional recipes. This spice combines well with almost any other ingredient, including banana. Cinnamon is considered to be a very beneficial spice, as it can help regulate healthy glucose levels in the blood, reduce pain linked to arthritis, and reduce LDL (bad) cholesterol levels.

- ⅓ cup melted butter, plus extra to grease loaf pan
- 1 cup granulated sugar, divided
- 1 large egg, beaten
- 2 teaspoons pure vanilla extract
- 3 large bananas, mashed
- 1½ cups gluten-free, all-purpose flour, plus extra to dust loaf pan
- 1 teaspoon baking soda
- Pinch of salt
- 1 tablespoon ground cinnamon

1. Preheat oven to 350 degrees F. Lightly grease a 9 x 5–inch loaf pan and dust with gluten-free flour.

2. In a medium bowl, blend together the butter, ¾ cup of the sugar, egg, and vanilla until well mixed. Add the mashed banana and stir to combine.

3. In a small bowl, toss together the flour, baking soda, and salt.

4. Add the dry ingredients to the wet ingredients, and stir to just combined—do not overmix.

5. In a small bowl, stir together the remaining sugar (¼ cup) and the cinnamon.

6. Spoon half the batter into the loaf pan, and then sprinkle about half of the cinnamon mixture over the batter.

7. Spoon the rest of the batter into the pan, and sprinkle the top with the remaining cinnamon mixture.

8. Run a knife through the batter a few times widthwise and lengthwise, and smooth the top again.

9. Bake for 50–60 minutes.

10. Let the loaf cool for 15 minutes. Then turn it out onto a wire rack until completely cool.

Makes 1 standard loaf (8–10 slices).

Walnut Date Bread

Walnuts are used quite regularly in quick breads because they have an almost meaty texture and a rich, fatty taste. Walnuts can also be slightly bitter and can become rancid quite easily. Always sample your walnuts before using them, or you might end up disappointed. If you can find them, black walnuts are a mild-tasting, sweeter choice.

- 1 cup almond flour
- ¼ cup coconut flour
- ½ teaspoon baking soda
- ¼ teaspoon sea salt
- 6 large Medjool dates, pitted
- 6 large eggs
- 2 tablespoons apple cider vinegar
- 1 cup chopped walnuts
- Coconut oil to grease loaf pans

1. Preheat oven to 350 degrees F and lightly grease two 2½ x 4½–inch mini loaf pans.

2. In a food processor, pulse together the almond flour, coconut flour, baking soda, and salt.

3. Add the dates to the processor and pulse until the mixture looks like crumbs.

4. Add the eggs and apple cider vinegar to the food processor and pulse to combine.

5. Add walnuts and pulse a couple of times.

6. Transfer the batter to the pans and smooth the tops.

7. Bake for 30–32 minutes, until a knife inserted in the center comes out clean.

8. Allow the bread to cool for at least 3 hours on a wire rack before removing the loaves from the pans.

Makes 2 small loaves (8–10 slices in total).

Double Chocolate Bread

This recipe looks long and complicated, but the results are worth it. There is a double dose of healthy dark chocolate in this bread, which nearly takes it out of the sweet bread category. Many experts recommend eating at least 1 ounce of dark chocolate each day because it is absolutely packed with antioxidants and many important minerals. It can also help promote a healthy cardiovascular system, assist in regulating blood sugar, and help fight many cancers.

- ¼ cup unsalted butter, at room temperature, plus extra to grease loaf pan
- 4 ounces chopped dark chocolate
- 2½ cups gluten-free, all-purpose flour, plus extra to dust loaf pan
- ½ cup granulated sugar
- ⅓ cup cocoa powder
- 1 tablespoon xanthan gum
- 1 tablespoon instant yeast
- 1 teaspoon baking soda
- ½ teaspoon sea salt
- ½ teaspoon ground cinnamon
- ½ teaspoon cream of tartar
- 1 tablespoon coconut oil
- 1 extra-large egg
- 1 extra-large egg white
- 1 teaspoon pure vanilla extract
- 1¼ cups almond milk, at about 100 degrees F
- 1 cup dark chocolate chips

1. Preheat oven to 350 degrees F. Lightly grease a 9 x 5–inch loaf pan and dust with flour.

2. Melt the butter and chopped dark chocolate in the microwave until smooth. Set aside.

3. In a large bowl, combine the flour, sugar, cocoa powder, xanthan gum, instant yeast, baking soda, sea salt, cinnamon, and cream of tartar until well blended.

4. Add the melted chocolate, oil, egg, egg white, and vanilla to the dry ingredients and beat until just moistened. Add the milk in a slow stream while beating. Add the chocolate chips and beat the dough for about 4 minutes.

5. Transfer the dough to the loaf pan and smooth the top.

6. Loosely cover the pan with plastic wrap, and place it in a warm spot until the dough rises about 1 inch above the top of the pan, about 1 hour.

7. Bake loaf for about 45 minutes until it is crusty and sounds hollow when tapped with your fingers.

8. Let the loaf cool for 15 minutes. Then turn it out onto a wire rack until completely cool.

Makes 1 standard loaf (8–10 slices).

Lemon Blueberry Bread

Fresh blueberries are the key to this sunny bread, so don't use frozen if you can avoid it. Frozen will work, but the texture and appearance of the bread will be different. Also, if you do use frozen berries, do not allow them to thaw before folding them into the batter.

For the bread:
- 1 cup plain yogurt
- 3 large eggs
- ⅓ cup coconut oil, plus extra to grease loaf pan
- ¼ cup finely grated lemon zest
- 1 teaspoon pure vanilla extract
- 1 cup granulated sugar
- ⅔ cup sorghum flour
- ⅓ cup brown rice flour, plus extra to dust loaf pan
- 1 tablespoon potato flour
- ⅓ cup cornstarch
- 2 tablespoons potato starch
- 1 tablespoon gluten-free baking powder
- ½ teaspoon xanthan gum
- ½ teaspoon salt
- 1½ cups fresh blueberries tossed with 1 tablespoon cornstarch

For the glaze:
- 1 cup powdered sugar
- 2½ tablespoons lemon juice

Make the bread:

1. Preheat oven to 350 degrees F. Lightly grease a 9 x 5–inch loaf pan and dust with rice flour.

2. In a large bowl, whisk together the yogurt, eggs, oil, zest, and vanilla.

3. In a medium bowl, whisk together the sugar, flours, cornstarch, potato starch, baking powder, xanthan gum, and salt.

4. Add the dry ingredients to the wet ingredients and stir to combine.

5. Fold the blueberries into the batter.

6. Spoon the batter into the loaf pan and bake 45–55 minutes, until a knife inserted in the center comes out clean.

7. Let the loaf cool for 15 minutes. Then turn it out onto a wire rack with foil or parchment paper underneath it.

Make the glaze:

8. Whisk together the powdered sugar and lemon juice until well blended.

9. Pour the glaze over the cooled loaf, and let it harden for at least 15 minutes before serving.

Makes 1 standard loaf (8–10 slices).

Simple Coconut Bread

You can throw this bread together quickly, yet it tastes like you slaved over it for hours. The flaked coconut provides a chewy texture and satisfying sweetness, while the almond milk is a perfect mix with the coconut flavor, especially if you choose an unsweetened product. Almond milk is one of the most nutritious dairy substitutes. It is an excellent source of vitamins A, D, E, and B, while being low in calories and sodium.

- 2½ cups gluten-free, all-purpose flour, plus extra to grease loaf pan
- 1 cup superfine sugar
- 1 tablespoon ground cinnamon
- 2 teaspoons gluten-free baking powder
- ½ teaspoon salt
- 1½ cups flaked coconut
- 2 large eggs
- 1¼ cups almond milk
- 1 teaspoon pure vanilla extract
- ⅓ cup unsalted butter, melted and cooled, plus extra to grease loaf pan

1. Preheat oven to 350 degrees F. Lightly grease a 8 x 4-inch loaf pan and dust with flour.

2. In a large bowl, stir together the flour, sugar, cinnamon, baking powder, and salt until well combined. Stir in the coconut.

3. In a small bowl, whisk together the eggs, milk, and vanilla until well blended.

4. Make a well in the center of the dry ingredients and pour in the egg mixture. Mix until just combined. Add the melted butter very carefully, folding it in until just combined.

5. Spoon the batter into the loaf pan.

6. Bake about 1 hour, until golden and a knife inserted in the center comes out clean.

7. Let the loaf cool for 10 minutes. Then turn it out onto a wire rack until completely cool.

Makes 1 small loaf (6–8 slices).

Nutella Banana Bread

Nutella is a much loved treat that just happens to be gluten-free—much to the delight of many people with gluten sensitivity. Nutella contains cocoa and hazelnuts, which combine beautifully with sweet banana. Hazelnuts are very high in vitamin E and essential linoleic acid, and they are 65 percent unsaturated fat. This loaf is a pretty marbled pattern, so you get a taste of banana and Nutella in each bite.

- 1 cup granulated sugar
- 4 tablespoons unsalted butter, at room temperature, plus extra to grease loaf pan
- 2 large eggs, lightly beaten
- 1 large ripe banana, mashed
- ⅓ cup plain yogurt
- 1 teaspoon pure vanilla extract
- 2 cups gluten-free, all-purpose flour
- ¾ teaspoon baking soda
- ½ teaspoon salt
- 1 cup Nutella

1. Preheat oven to 350 degrees F and lightly grease an 8 x 4–inch loaf pan.

2. In a large bowl, beat together the sugar and butter until creamy. Add the eggs, mashed banana, yogurt, and vanilla and beat to blend well.

3. In a small bowl, stir together the flour, baking soda, and salt and add to the banana mixture, stirring just until combined.

4. Place the Nutella in a bowl and microwave on low heat until soft.

5. Add about 1 cup of the batter to the Nutella and stir to combine.

6. Spoon the batters into the loaf pan, alternating between the plain banana and the Nutella.

7. Run a sharp knife through the batter a couple of times to swirl.

8. Bake the bread for 50–60 minutes, until a knife inserted in the center comes out clean.

9. Let the loaf cool for 10 minutes. Then turn it out onto a wire rack until completely cool.

Makes 1 small loaf (6–8 slices).

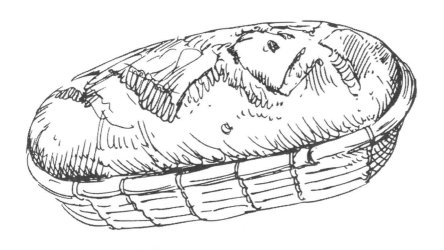

Bread is the warmest, kindest of all words. Write it always with a capital letter, like your own name.

—Anonymous

4

FLATBREADS, MUFFINS, PIZZA DOUGH, AND MORE

Cheesy Breadsticks

The best way to create these breadsticks is with a large piping bag, but if you don't have one, you can also fill a large freezer bag with your batter. Then you simply cut a hole in one corner and squeeze the dough out in a steady stream. The size of the hole will determine the width of your breadsticks, so try to make the hole about ¾ of an inch.

- 1 cup sorghum flour
- ⅔ cup potato starch
- ⅓ cup tapioca flour
- 2 tablespoons granulated sugar
- 1½ tablespoons xanthan gum
- 1 teaspoon salt
- 1 tablespoon instant yeast
- 1 cup warm almond milk (105–115 degrees F)
- ⅓ cup grated Parmesan cheese
- 2 tablespoons extra-virgin olive oil
- 1 teaspoon apple cider vinegar
- Coconut oil to grease cookie sheet and brush breadsticks

98

1. Lightly grease a cookie sheet.

2. In a large bowl, combine the sorghum flour, potato starch, tapioca flour, sugar, xanthan gum, salt, and instant yeast until well mixed.

3. In a medium bowl, stir together the almond milk, Parmesan cheese, olive oil, and apple cider vinegar.

4. Add the wet ingredients to the dry ingredients and beat for several minutes until combined.

5. Place the batter in a large piping bag topped with just the coupler.

6. Squeeze the dough onto the cookie sheet, holding the bag upright.

7. Brush the tops of the breadsticks with coconut oil.

8. Turn the oven to 400 degrees F, and place the breadsticks into the cold oven as it heats up.

9. Bake for about 20 minutes, until lightly browned.

Makes 12 breadsticks.

Sun-Dried Tomato and Herb Flatbread

Flatbread is a versatile treat that can be used as a base for a light lunch, a snack in the afternoon, or an accompaniment to a satisfying stew or soup. This flatbread would be spectacular grilled with a fresh green salad on a balmy summer night. Garbanzo bean flour is not a commonly found ingredient, but it is worthwhile to source it out. It is very nutritious, is high in fiber and protein, and does not have to be combined with other flours to create a nice product.

- 2 cups garbanzo bean flour
- 1¾ cups quinoa flour
- ¾ cup almond flour
- 1 tablespoon sea salt
- 2 cups warm-to-hot water
- 2 large eggs, beaten
- 2 teaspoons baking soda
- 1 teaspoon apple cider vinegar
- ¾ cup chopped sun-dried tomatoes
- 1 teaspoon chopped fresh basil
- 1 teaspoon chopped fresh rosemary
- Extra-virgin olive oil to grease cookie sheet

1. Preheat oven to 400 degrees F and lightly grease a cookie sheet.

2. In a large bowl, stir together the garbanzo bean flour, quinoa flour, almond flour, salt, and water until relatively smooth and let sit on the counter until the mixture cools to lukewarm.

3. Add the eggs, baking soda, and apple cider vinegar, and stir to combine.

4. Let the dough rise for about 15 minutes and then fold in the tomatoes and herbs.

5. Transfer the batter to the cookie sheet, smoothing it into a rough rectangle.

6. Bake for 25–30 minutes, until browned.

7. Let the flatbread cool for 10–15 minutes before serving.

Makes 16 slices.

Airy Herb Popovers

If you have never tried popovers, this recipe will be a great introduction. The most important part of this baking process is to preheat the muffin pan in the oven before spooning in the batter. If you skip this step, your popovers will not be hollow and slightly creamy in the center. These golden treats are a little like Yorkshire pudding and can be used alongside prime rib with great success.

- 4 large eggs
- 1 cup almond milk
- ⅔ cup rice flour
- ⅓ cup tapioca flour
- 2 teaspoons chopped fresh thyme

- 1 teaspoon chopped fresh rosemary
- 1 teaspoon chopped fresh oregano
- Pinch of sea salt
- Cooking spray for the muffin tin

---

1. Preheat oven to 425 degrees F, and place a 12-cup muffin pan in the oven while it is heating up.

2. In a large bowl, beat together the eggs and milk until very well blended.

3. Add the rice flour, tapioca flour, herbs, and salt, and whisk until the batter is smooth.

4. Remove the heated muffin pan from the oven carefully, and spray it lightly with the cooking spray.

5. Spoon the batter into each cup, filling them about three-quarters of the way full.

6. Bake for about 20–25 minutes, until golden and puffed. Serve immediately.

Makes 12 popovers.

Gluten-Free Bagels

This recipe does not produce a perfect bagel, but it is a pretty good gluten-free substitute. These have a muffinlike texture but can be sliced easily once they are completely cool. You can leave out the raisins and add chocolate chips depending on your taste preference, and try them toasted with a little almond butter or homemade jam for a real treat.

- ¼ cup almond milk
- ¼ cup melted coconut oil, plus extra to grease cookie sheet
- ¼ cup unsweetened applesauce
- 3 tablespoons flaxseed meal
- 2 tablespoons water
- 1 tablespoon pure maple syrup
- 2 teaspoons apple cider vinegar
- ¾ teaspoon xanthan gum
- ½ cup coconut flour
- ½ cup tapioca flour
- 2 teaspoons ground cinnamon
- 1 teaspoon baking soda
- 1 teaspoon gluten-free baking powder
- ¼ cup raisins

1. Preheat oven to 350 degrees F and lightly grease a cookie sheet.

2. In a large bowl, beat together the almond milk, coconut oil, applesauce, flaxseed meal, water, maple syrup, apple cider vinegar, and xanthan gum until well combined.

3. In a small bowl, stir together the flours, cinnamon, baking soda, baking powder, and raisins until well combined.

4. Add the dry ingredients to the wet ingredients, and stir until incorporated and a dough ball starts to form.

5. Divide the dough into four equal parts and roll each piece into a ball. Poke your finger through the center of each ball to create a bagel shape.

6. Bake for 20–25 minutes, until golden. Let the bagels cool completely and then chill before slicing.

Makes 4 bagels.

Tempting Blueberry Muffins

This is a sweet, cakelike muffin that is absolutely bursting with blueberries. You can substitute pretty much any fruit in this almond-scented batter with delicious results. So try ripe peaches, red raspberries, cherries, apricots, and even apples for different variations. Add a little more honey if your fruit isn't completely ripe.

- 2 cups almond flour
- ¼ teaspoon baking soda
- ⅛ teaspoon sea salt
- 1 cup full-fat coconut milk
- 2 large eggs
- ¼ cup honey
- ¼ cup melted coconut oil
- ¾ cup fresh blueberries

1. Preheat oven to 350 degrees F and line a 12-cup muffin pan with paper liners.

2. In a large bowl, stir together the almond flour, baking soda, and salt until well mixed.

3. In a medium bowl, stir together the coconut milk, eggs, honey, and coconut oil until well blended.

4. Add the wet ingredients to the almond flour mixture and stir to combine.

5. Fold the blueberries into the batter carefully.

6. Spoon the batter into the muffin cups and bake for 20–25 minutes, until golden brown.

7. Let the muffins cool completely before removing them from the pan.

Makes 12 muffins.

Autumn Dinner Rolls

Pumpkin puree makes these golden rolls a lovely addition to a Thanksgiving or Christmas dinner table. There is just enough pumpkin to impart moisture and sweetness without losing the almost buttery taste. This recipe can be doubled easily if your gathering is large or you want to freeze some rolls to enjoy later.

- 3 large eggs
- ½ cup pumpkin puree (canned or freshly roasted)
- 2 cups almond flour, plus extra to dust dough balls
- ¼ cup coconut flour
- 2 tablespoons melted coconut oil, plus extra to grease loaf pan
- 1 tablespoon water, plus extra if necessary

1. Preheat oven to 400 degrees F and lightly grease a 9-inch round cake pan.

2. In a medium bowl, using an electric mixer, beat the eggs until light yellow and frothy. Add the pumpkin puree and stir until well combined.

3. In a large bowl, stir together the almond flour, coconut flour, and coconut oil until well combined. Stir in the water.

4. Add the egg mixture to the flour mixture and stir until well combined.

5. Allow the dough to rest for 5 minutes and then stir again, adding a little more water if necessary to make the dough pliable and easy to knead. The dough should be lightly sticky, but not wet. Allow the dough to rest for 5 more minutes.

6. Divide the dough into 12 equal pieces. Lightly knead each piece of dough into a ball, dusting with some almond flour to keep the dough soft. Transfer the dough rolls into the cake pan.

7. Bake for 20–25 minutes, until the tops of the rolls are browned. Cool completely before serving.

Makes 12 rolls.

Buttermilk Biscuits

These are traditional Southern-style biscuits made with very few ingredients and real buttermilk. Buttermilk sounds like it should be very fattening and unhealthy, but it is actually low in fat because it has been removed from the butter-making process. Buttermilk is a great source of phosphorus, calcium, potassium, and vitamin B_{12}. It imparts a pleasing, tart taste to baked products and produces a tender texture.

- 6 large egg whites
- ½ cup buttermilk
- ¼ teaspoon apple cider vinegar
- 1½ cups almond flour
- ¼ cup coconut flour
- 2 teaspoons gluten-free baking powder
- 2 tablespoons chilled coconut oil

---

1. Preheat the oven to 350 degrees F and line a baking sheet with parchment paper.

2. In a medium bowl, using an electric mixer, beat the egg whites, buttermilk, and apple cider vinegar until well combined.

3. In a large bowl, stir together the almond flour, coconut flour, and baking powder until combined. Add the cold coconut oil and mix with a fork until the mixture resembles coarse crumbs.

4. Add the egg mixture to the dry ingredients and stir until a wet dough forms.

5. Using an ice-cream scoop, scoop rounded portions of the dough onto the baking sheet. Bake for 10–15 minutes, until the tops of the biscuits are lightly browned. Allow the biscuits to cool for a few minutes before serving.

Makes 8 biscuits.

Rosemary Flatbread

The technique used to make flatbread is as simple as spreading the dough out on a cookie sheet and baking it to a crispy, golden brown. This is a good recipe just to try out gluten-free bread baking if you are new to this type of diet. The almond butter in this recipe can be replaced with cashew butter if you want a slightly richer, denser bread.

- ¼ cup almond flour
- ¼ cup arrowroot powder
- 1 teaspoon baking soda
- ¾ cup raw almond butter
- 1 tablespoon raw honey
- 3 large eggs
- 2 tablespoons finely chopped rosemary
- 3 tablespoons extra-virgin olive oil
- Coarse sea salt for topping (optional)

1. Preheat oven to 350 degrees F and line a 9 x 13–inch jelly-roll pan with parchment paper.

2. In a small bowl, stir together the almond flour, arrowroot powder, and baking soda until combined.

3. In a large bowl, combine the almond butter and honey. Add the eggs, one at a time, stirring between each addition. Stir in the rosemary.

4. Add the flour mixture to the wet ingredients and stir until a wet dough forms.

5. Drizzle the olive oil on the parchment-lined jelly-roll pan and spread the dough over it. Allow the dough to rest for 5 minutes.

6. Bake for 25–30 minutes, until the top of the bread is golden brown.

7. Top with sea salt if desired. Allow the bread to cool.

Makes 12 servings.

Sweet Cinnamon Rolls

Most people avoid making cinnamon rolls because the process looks quite complicated. This is not the case with this recipe because there is no yeast involved. The most difficult step is usually cutting the rolls, but that can also be simple if you use dental floss or even fishing line. If you plan on making a lot of these delicious treats, make a permanent cutter by knotting a length of floss between two dowels.

For the dough:

- 2 large eggs
- 1 tablespoon raw honey
- ¼ cup coconut oil plus 2 tablespoons, divided
- 2 cups almond flour
- 1 teaspoon baking soda
- 2 tablespoons ground cinnamon
- 3 tablespoons coconut sugar
- ½ cup coarsely chopped pecans

For the icing:

- ¼ cup full-fat canned coconut milk
- ¼ cup coconut sugar
- 1 tablespoon pure vanilla extract
- 1 teaspoon arrowroot powder

Make the dough:

1. Preheat oven to 350 degrees F.

2. In a large bowl, using an electric mixer, beat the eggs and honey. Add ¼ cup of coconut oil and stir to combine.

3. In a medium bowl, stir together the almond flour and baking soda.

4. Add the flour mixture to the wet ingredients, and stir until a stiff dough forms.

5. Lay a large piece of parchment paper on a clean surface and place the dough on it. Lay another piece of parchment on top,

and then roll out the dough until you have a rectangle about ¼-inch thick.

6. In a small bowl, combine the 2 tablespoons of coconut oil, cinnamon, and sugar. Sprinkle over the rolled-out dough. Then sprinkle with the chopped pecans.

7. Roll up the dough, starting with the longer side of the rectangle, and slice into eight to ten (2-inch thick) cinnamon rolls. Position the rolls on a parchment-paper-lined baking sheet.

8. Bake for 15–20 minutes, until the rolls are lightly browned.

Make the icing:

9. In a small bowl, stir together the coconut milk, sugar, vanilla, and arrowroot powder until well combined.

10. Using a spoon or spatula, drizzle the icing over the warm cinnamon rolls and serve warm.

Makes about 8–10 rolls.

Golden Breadsticks

Fresh garlic is the key to the spectacular flavor of these crispy creations. Garlic is a member of the onion family. It has a well-deserved reputation for being an herbal cure because it is a natural antibiotic and antioxidant. Studies have shown it helps the body fight free radicals and promotes a healthy immune system while boosting the ability to fight cancer, heart disease, and hypertension. Do not replace the fresh garlic in the recipe with powdered garlic because that will change the flavor and mute the health benefits.

For the breadsticks:

- 1½ cups almond flour
- 1 teaspoon dried oregano
- ½ teaspoon dried basil
- ½ teaspoon sea salt
- ¼ teaspoon minced garlic
- 1 tablespoon extra-virgin olive oil
- 2 large eggs, beaten
- 2 tablespoons coconut flour, divided

For the topping:

- 1 large egg
- 1 teaspoon water
- ½ teaspoon dried basil
- ½ teaspoon sea salt
- ¼ teaspoon garlic powder

Make the breadsticks:

1. Preheat oven to 350 degrees F.

2. In a medium bowl, stir together almond flour, oregano, basil, sea salt, garlic, olive oil, and eggs until combined. Let the dough set for several minutes, and then add about 1 tablespoon of the coconut flour, stirring to mix.

3. Let the dough sit again so the coconut flour can dry it out, and then add the remaining 1 tablespoon of coconut flour. Stir to combine, and roll the dough into a ball. Divide the ball into four equal pieces.

4. On a clean work surface, roll one piece of dough into a long snake about ½-inch thick. Fold the snake in half so there are two equal pieces the same length lying side by side.

5. Pinch the two ends together on both ends, and twist the two pieces together carefully to form a twisty rope. Place on a parchment-paper-lined baking sheet. Repeat with the remaining pieces.

6. Bake for about 10 minutes and then remove from the oven.

Make the topping:
7. While the breadsticks are baking, whisk together the egg and water in a small bowl.

8. In a small cup, toss together the basil, sea salt, and garlic powder.

9. Once the breadsticks have been removed from the oven (see step 6), flip them over with a spatula.

10. Brush the tops of the breadsticks with the egg wash, and then sprinkle with the herb mix.

11. Return the breadsticks to the oven and bake for an additional 5 minutes. Allow the breadsticks to cool for 2–5 minutes before serving.

Makes 4 breadsticks.

Soft Pretzels

This is a great recipe to make with kids because it is fun to twist the dough into pretzel shapes. You might end up with some interesting-looking pretzels, but they will still taste wonderful topped with a pretty sprinkle of coarse sea salt. Pretzels are perfect lunch-bag stuffers and treats to tote on long car rides because they are healthier than fatty chips or sugary cookies, but they still taste like a snack food.

- ½ cup extra-virgin olive oil, plus extra to brush pretzels
- ½ cup of water
- 2 tablespoons apple cider vinegar
- 2 teaspoons of sea salt, divided

- ½ cup of tapioca flour
- ½ teaspoon gluten-free baking powder
- ½ teaspoon baking soda
- 1 cup coconut flour
- 1 large egg, lightly beaten

1. Preheat oven to 350 degrees F.

2. Place the olive oil, water, apple cider vinegar, and ½ teaspoon of the salt in a medium saucepan, and bring to a boil over medium heat.

3. Remove from the heat and add the tapioca flour. Stir to combine. Add the baking powder and baking soda to the mixture and stir. The mixture will foam. Add the coconut flour and egg, and mix until a firm dough forms.

4. Turn the dough out onto a work surface lightly dusted with tapioca flour, and knead the dough for 2–5 minutes.

5. Pinch off a 2-inch piece of dough, and roll it into a thin snake about 6 inches long. Twist the log into a traditional pretzel

shape. (This might take a little practice.) Place the pretzel on a parchment-paper-lined baking sheet. Repeat until all the dough is used up.

6. Brush the pretzels with a little olive oil, and sprinkle sea salt over them. Bake for 25–30 minutes, until golden. Serve warm whenever possible.

Makes about 18 pretzels.

Perfect Pizza Dough

Many people dream of pizza and are very concerned about this dish when finding out they need to start a gluten-free diet. This recipe produces a very nice, thin crust that can be topped with all your favorite pizza choices. You can create a thicker crust if that is your preference by not pressing out the dough too thin. If your crust is thicker, you might want to prebake it for about 10 minutes before putting the toppings on to make sure it cooks through.

- 1⅔ cups almond flour
- ½ cup arrowroot powder
- 2 teaspoons minced garlic
- ½ teaspoon baking soda
- 1 teaspoon sea salt
- 2 large eggs

- 4 teaspoons extra-virgin olive oil
- 1 teaspoon chopped fresh rosemary
- 1 teaspoon chopped fresh oregano

---

1. Preheat oven to 350 degrees F.

2. In a large bowl, stir together the almond flour, arrowroot powder, garlic, baking soda, and salt.

3. In a small bowl, whisk the eggs and oil together with the herbs.

4. Add the wet ingredients to the dry ingredients, and mix well until the batter forms into a ball. Add more almond flour if the dough is too wet.

5. Press the dough onto a 12-inch pizza pan, or form a rough circle on a cookie sheet. Crimp the edges slightly to create a lip all the way around.

6. Top with desired toppings and bake for about 20 minutes or until crisp.

Makes a 12-inch pizza crust.

Pumpkin Scones

This might become the new family favorite for breakfast and a tempting snack when you need a bit of an energy lift. To get the finest tender texture, rather than a biscuit-style creation, make sure you do not overwork the butter. The butter should be very cold, and the pieces not too large when rubbing it into the dry ingredients. If the butter melts due to the heat of your hands, there will not be tiny pockets of buttery goodness in the dough. You can also use a fork instead of your fingers for this step if you naturally have warm hands.

For the scones:

- 2 cups gluten-free, all-purpose flour
- 7 tablespoons granulated sugar
- 2 teaspoons gluten-free baking powder
- 1½ teaspoons pumpkin pie spice
- ½ teaspoon salt
- ⅓ cup cold butter, cut into 1-inch cubes
- ½ cup pumpkin puree
- ¼ cup almond milk
- 1 large egg

For the glaze:

- 1 cup confectioner's sugar
- 2 tablespoons almond milk
- ½ teaspoon ground cinnamon
- ⅓ teaspoon ground nutmeg
- Dash of ground cloves

Make the scones:

1. Preheat the oven to 425 degrees F and line a baking sheet with parchment paper.

2. In a large bowl, mix together the flour, sugar, baking powder, pumpkin pie spice, and salt until well combined. Add the cubed butter and rub it in using your fingertips until the dough resembles crumbs.

3. Stir in the pumpkin puree, almond milk, and egg, and stir to combine.

4. Gather the dough together, and press it into a large square shape on a lightly floured surface.

5. Cut the dough into four smaller squares, and then cut an X pattern (4 pieces) in each square portion to get sixteen triangular pieces of dough.

6. Place the scones on the baking sheet, and bake for about 15 minutes, until golden.

7. Cool the scones on wire rack for 10 minutes.

Make the glaze:
8. In a medium bowl, whisk all the ingredients together until smooth.

9. When the scones are cool, pick them up and dip the tops into the glaze. Put them back on the wire rack and let stand for about 1 hour, until the glaze hardens.

Makes 16 scones.

Potato Focaccia Bread

Potato is an ingredient you don't see every day in breads, but there is actually a fine history behind the addition of this starchy star. Traditional potato bread actually uses potato to replace some of the bulk of wheat flour in a recipe, so it is perfect for gluten-free concoctions. These simple rustic breads can be found in many countries such as Ireland, Scotland, Germany, Poland, and the United States.

- 1 cup warm water (about 110–115 degrees F)
- 1 tablespoon granulated sugar
- 1 tablespoon active dry yeast
- 1 cup sorghum flour
- ¾ cup tapioca flour
- ½ cup sweet rice flour
- ⅔ cup potato starch
- 1½ teaspoons xanthan gum
- 1 teaspoon sea salt
- 1 large egg, separated
- ¼ cup extra-virgin olive oil, plus extra to grease pie pan and sprinkle on dough
- 1 tablespoon finely chopped fresh rosemary
- 1 large potato, peeled, cooked in heavily salted water, and mashed

1. In a small bowl, stir together the warm water and sugar. Sprinkle the yeast over the water and let it stand until it gets foamy, about 10 minutes.

2. In a large bowl, stir together the flours, potato starch, xanthan gum, and salt until well combined.

3. Add the egg yolk, oil, rosemary, yeast mixture, and mashed potato to the dry ingredients. Stir until the dough comes together, about 5 minutes.

4. In a small bowl, whisk the egg white until stiff peaks form.

5. Fold the egg white into the dough, and set aside in a warm spot for about 1 hour or until it doubles in size.

6. Preheat the oven to 450 degrees F and place a piece of parchment paper in a 9-inch pie pan. Grease the paper generously.

7. Transfer the dough to the pan and smooth the top.

8. Sprinkle top with olive oil and bake for about 25 minutes, until the top is browned.

9. Cool in the pan for 10 minutes and then remove it. Cool for about 15 minutes more and serve.

Makes 1 medium focaccia (4 servings).

Pumpkin Cinnamon Rolls

This recipe is a bit more complicated than popping premade cinnamon rolls in a pan and baking them. However, the finished bread is scrumptious and well worth the time it takes to make them. You can use plain icing for the glaze instead of the pumpkin variation, but the extra pumpkin flavor really picks up the taste in the rolls and elevates these cinnamon-scented rolls to something truly sublime.

For the pumpkin rolls:
- ⅓ cup warm almond milk (110–115 degrees F)
- ¾ cup granulated sugar
- 2 tablespoons active dry yeast
- ⅔ cup canned pumpkin puree
- ¼ cup extra-virgin olive oil, plus extra to grease pans
- 1 teaspoon pure vanilla extract
- ¾ cup tapioca starch
- ½ cup sorghum flour
- ¼ cup brown rice flour
- ½ cup cornstarch
- 1 tablespoon gluten-free baking powder
- 2 teaspoons xanthan gum
- ½ teaspoon baking soda
- ½ teaspoon sea salt

For the filling:
- 4 tablespoons packed brown sugar
- 2 tablespoons ground cinnamon
- 6 tablespoons unsalted butter, at room temperature

For the icing:
- ¼ cup pumpkin puree
- 2 tablespoons room-temperature butter
- 3½ cups powdered sugar

To make the rolls:

1. Lightly grease four round 8-inch cake pans.

2. In a small bowl, combine the almond milk and sugar. Sprinkle the yeast on top and set aside until foamy, about 10 minutes.

3. Stir in the pumpkin puree, olive oil, and vanilla into the yeast mixture, and set aside.

4. In a large bowl, stir together the tapioca starch, flours, cornstarch, baking powder, xanthan gum, baking soda, and salt until well mixed.

5. Add the yeast mixture to the dry ingredients until an elastic sticky dough is formed.

6. Turn the dough out onto a lightly oiled piece of parchment paper and pat into a rectangle shape.

Make the filling:

7. In a small, bowl toss together the brown sugar and cinnamon.

8. Spread the softened butter over the dough and sprinkle evenly with the sugar mixture.

9. Carefully roll the dough into a long cylinder, using the parchment to help.

10. Slice the cinnamon rolls using a sharp knife or dental floss, and place the rolls into the pans, leaving about 1 inch between the rolls.

11. Cover the pans loosely with plastic wrap, and let rise in a warm place for about 45 minutes.

12. Preheat oven to 350 degrees F.

13. Bake rolls for 30–35 minutes.

14. Cool on wire rack.

Make the pumpkin icing:

15. In a medium bowl, cream together the pumpkin and butter until smooth.

16. Add the powdered sugar until icing is spreadable and sweet to taste.

17. Frost rolls generously with icing.

Makes 16 rolls.

Chocolate Peanut Butter Muffins

Reese's Peanut Butter Cups are a perennial favorite in many households, and this muffin tastes very close to those delectable little bites. Peanut butter is usually considered to be fattening and unhealthy; however, it contains unsaturated fat (mostly), folate, niacin (vitamin B₃), protein, dietary fiber, and resveratrol. This means this creamy treat can help reduce the risk of heart disease, increase the level of good cholesterol, and help fight cancer.

- ½ cup butter
- ½ cup honey
- 1 cup peanut butter
- ½ cup cocoa powder
- 4 large eggs, lightly beaten
- ½ teaspoon baking soda
- 1 cup dark chocolate chips

1. Preheat oven to 350 degrees F and line a 12-cup muffin pan with paper liners.

2. In a large saucepan over low heat, melt the butter and honey together.

3. Remove from heat and whisk in the peanut butter until smooth.

4. Stir in the cocoa powder until well incorporated.

5. Add the eggs and baking soda, and stir to combine well.

6. Stir in the chocolate chips and spoon the batter into the muffin cups evenly.

7. Bake for 20–22 minutes, until a toothpick inserted in the center comes out clean.

Makes 12 muffins.

Baking-Powder Biscuits

Biscuits are a breeze to make and can be thoroughly addictive eaten warm (even hot!) from the oven. Baking-powder biscuits actually have a firm place in culinary history because many people did not have ovens or stoves that could be used for bread making. These types of biscuits were made instead, baked fresh with very few ingredients. This gluten-free variation has a few more ingredients, but it is still fabulous served piping hot like their colonial cousins.

- 3½ cups gluten-free, all-purpose flour, plus extra for rolling
- ½ cup granulated sugar
- 1 tablespoon xanthan gum
- 2½ teaspoons gluten-free baking powder
- ¼ teaspoon sea salt
- ¾ cup chilled and cubed unsalted butter
- 2 large eggs, lightly beaten
- 1 cup cold whole milk, plus 2 tablespoons more to brush biscuits
- ½ cup brown sugar mixed with 1 teaspoon ground cinnamon

1. Preheat oven to 350 degrees F and place a sheet of parchment paper on a baking sheet.

2. In a large bowl, stir together the flour, sugar, xanthan gum, baking powder, and salt until well combined.

3. Add the cold butter and rub the mixture between your fingertips until it resembles coarse crumbs.

4. Make a well in the center of the butter mixture, and add the eggs and milk. Toss until mixture comes together.

5. Turn the dough out onto a lightly floured surface, and press dough into a disk.

6. Sprinkle flour on top of the disk, and roll the dough out so it is a rough rectangle about ¾-inch thick.

7. Fold the edges over each other like a letter and roll out again to about ¾-inch thick. Cut out 3-inch round biscuits using a water glass or cutter, and place them about 1 inch apart on the baking sheet.

8. Place the baking sheet in the freezer for about 10 minutes.

9. Take the sheet out and brush the tops of the chilled biscuits with milk. Sprinkle with the brown sugar mixture.

10. Bake for about 20 minutes, until golden brown.

11. Allow to cool about 5 minutes before serving toasty warm.

Makes 12 biscuits.

Pear Almond Muffins

These are a moist, vanilla-scented treat that is satisfying in their simplicity of taste and preparation. Try them with a steaming cup of herbal tea for breakfast, or pack one in a child's lunch to provide a healthy energy source for an action-packed day. The brown sugar and spice create a lightly caramelized finish that might make you crave more than one!

- 2¼ cups almond flour
- 1 teaspoon ground cinnamon
- ½ teaspoon salt
- ¼ teaspoon gluten-free baking powder
- 1 large egg
- ¼ cup almond milk
- ¼ cup honey
- ¼ cup melted coconut oil
- 1 teaspoon pure vanilla extract
- ½ teaspoon baking soda
- 1 cup grated pear
- ½ cup sliced almonds
- 2 tablespoons brown sugar mixed with ½ teaspoon cinnamon

---

1. Preheat oven to 375 degrees F and line a 9-cup muffin pan with paper liners.

2. In a large bowl, stir together the almond flour, cinnamon, salt, and baking powder until well combined.

3. In a medium bowl, whisk together the egg, almond milk, honey, oil, vanilla, and baking soda.

4. Add the wet ingredients to the dry ingredients, and stir until just combined.

5. Fold in the grated pear and almonds.

6. Spoon the muffin batter into the prepared muffin cups, filling them nearly to the top.

7. Sprinkle the muffin tops with the brown sugar mixture and bake for about 15 minutes, until muffins are browned and a toothpick inserted in the center comes out clean.

8. Let the muffins cool in the pan for 5 minutes, before removing them and cooling completely on a wire rack.

Makes 9 muffins.

Morning Glory Muffins

Morning glory muffins were originally introduced to muffin lovers in Gourmet magazine back in 1981 by Chef Pam McKinstry. Ten years later, they were voted in the top 25 recipes ever in the magazine, and countless recipes have been created since as a tribute to the original—like these gluten-free gems. These muffins are actually better the second day after the flavors mellow, so try to store them overnight if there are any left.

- 1 cup sorghum flour
- ½ cup gluten-free oats
- 2 teaspoon gluten-free baking powder
- 1 teaspoon ground cinnamon
- ½ teaspoon ground nutmeg
- ½ teaspoon sea salt
- ¼ teaspoon ground cloves
- 2 large eggs
- 1 cup unsweetened applesauce
- ½ cup melted coconut oil
- ¼ cup honey
- 1 tablespoon pure vanilla extract
- 2 cups finely grated carrot
- ¾ cup shredded unsweetened coconut
- ½ cup organic raisins
- ⅓ cup chopped pecans

1. Preheat oven to 350 degrees F and line a 12-cup muffin pan with paper liners.

2. In a medium bowl, stir together the flour, oats, baking powder, cinnamon, nutmeg, sea salt, and cloves until well combined.

3. In a large bowl, whisk together the eggs, applesauce, coconut oil, honey, and vanilla.

4. Add the dry ingredients to the wet ingredients and stir to combine.

5. Stir in the grated carrot, coconut, raisins, and pecans.

6. Spoon the batter into the muffin pan, filling each cup close to the top.

7. Bake for 30–35 minutes, until a toothpick inserted in the center comes out clean.

8. Cool for at least 15 minutes before serving.

Makes 12 muffins.

Gluten-Free Crumpets

Crumpets are sometimes confused with English muffins. The difference can lie in the ingredients, and most often, in the appearance of this bread. Crumpets have a flat, toasted bottom with a pale top covered in holes, while English muffins are cooked on both sides. This gluten-free recipe breaks a few ingredient rules associated with crumpets, but the finished product is traditional in appearance.

- 1 cup gluten-free, all-purpose flour
- 1 tablespoon granulated sugar
- 1 teaspoon active dry yeast
- Pinch of salt
- 1 cup almond milk
- 2 tablespoons melted butter, plus extra to grease crumpet rings

1. Lightly grease four crumpet rings and a skillet.

2. In a large bowl, stir together the flour, sugar, yeast, and salt until well mixed.

3. Add the almond milk and melted butter to the dry ingredients, and stir until smooth.

4. Cover the bowl with plastic wrap and place in a warm location until risen, about 1–1½ hours. Stir down the batter.

5. Heat the greased skillet over medium-high heat, and place the crumpet rings in the skillet.

6. Reduce heat to low, pour about ⅓ cup of batter into each crumpet ring, and cook over low heat for about 5 minutes, until the batter looks like it is filled with holes.

7. Use tongs to remove the crumpet rings, and flip the crumpets over. Cook about 5 minutes more.

8. Repeat this process until the batter is used up.

Makes 10–12 crumpets.

Pull-Apart Honey Rolls

These rolls can be whipped up for a special breakfast with a little planning and the help of a heavy-duty mixer. They are sweet without being cloying and can be eaten without the glaze if you want a simpler version.

For the rolls:

- 4–4½ cups gluten-free, all-purpose flour
- 2 tablespoons active dry yeast
- 3 teaspoons xanthan gum
- ½ teaspoon salt
- ¼ teaspoon cream of tartar
- ½ cup grapeseed oil
- 2 tablespoons honey
- 1 extra-large egg

- 1 extra-large egg white
- 2 cups warm almond milk (between 100–115 degrees F)

For the glaze:

- ½ cup brown sugar
- 2 tablespoons melted and cooled unsalted butter
- 1 tablespoon honey
- 1 extra-large egg

Make the rolls:

1. Place parchment paper in two 8 x 8–inch baking pans.

2. In a large bowl, combine the flour, yeast, xanthan gum, salt, and cream of tartar until well blended.

3. Make a well in the center of the dry ingredients, and add the oil, honey, egg, and egg white into the center. Mix until incorporated.

4. Add the milk to the batter, and beat for about 5 minutes until the dough is thick and smooth.

5. Lightly flour a work surface and turn the dough out. Divide the dough into twenty-four equal balls, and place twelve in each baking pan, spaced evenly.

6. Cover the pans with plastic and place them in a warm place to rise for about 30–45 minutes, until they have almost doubled in size and are touching each other.

7. Preheat oven to 375 degrees F.

Make the glaze:

8. Mix all the glaze ingredients in a small bowl, and brush the tops of the risen buns generously with the glaze.

9. Bake buns for 18–20 minutes, until lightly browned.

10. Cool for about 10 minutes and serve warm.

Makes 24 buns.

Tortillas

Tortillas can be rolled around an assortment of tempting fillings, and this recipe is simple and tasty. You must roll the tortillas out very thin to get pliable rounds that will actually wrap rather than crack. You can add a touch of thyme, cayenne, or cumin to this batter for different variations.

- 2 cups almond flour
- 2 large eggs, lightly beaten
- 1 teaspoon melted coconut oil
- ¼ teaspoon salt (or to taste)
- Water, if needed
- 3 tablespoons extra-virgin olive oil, or as needed for frying

1. Combine the almond flour, eggs, coconut oil, and salt in a medium bowl until well mixed.

2. Gather the dough into a ball and knead using the sides of the bowl until the dough is elastic. Add a little water if the dough is too dry.

3. Divide the dough in four to six equal balls, and roll out each ball thinly between two pieces of parchment paper.

4. Heat the olive oil in a frying pan over medium heat and fry each tortilla, turning once until cooked, about 30 seconds a side.

5. Remove tortillas from the pan and place on paper towels to drain.

6. Repeat until all the tortillas are cooked.

7. Serve warm, wrapped around a favorite filling.

Makes 4–6 tortillas, depending on the size.

Hamburger Buns

The dough in this recipe is quite soft and a little hard to work with, but the finished buns could pass easily for their wheat-loaded cousins. You must make sure that your hands are oiled when rolling the buns into rounds or the dough will stick too much to be workable. Don't forget to sprinkle the tops with sesame seeds to create a truly authentic look.

- 2½ cups gluten-free, all-purpose flour
- ½ cup confectioner's sugar
- ⅓ cup whey powder
- 2 teaspoons gluten-free baking powder
- 2 teaspoons xanthan gum
- ½ teaspoon sea salt

- ¼ teaspoon cream of tartar
- 5 extra-large eggs
- ⅔ cup melted and cooled unsalted butter
- ½ cup, at room temperature almond milk
- ¾ teaspoon apple cider vinegar

---

1. Preheat oven to 375 degrees F and line two baking sheets with parchment paper.

2. In a large bowl, stir together the flour, confectioner's sugar, whey powder, baking powder, xanthan gum, salt, and cream of tartar until well combined.

3. Add the eggs, butter, almond milk, and apple cider vinegar, and beat until the batter is very well blended, pale, and thick.

4. Using wet hands, divide the dough into twelve equal parts. Form into rounds and then flatten them out to about 1-inch thick. Place on the baking sheets about 2 inches apart.

5. Bake for 15 minutes and then rotate the trays. Lower the oven temperature to 325 degrees F, and bake for an additional 30

minutes. After 15 minutes, rotate the trays again, and cut a slit in the tops of the buns to allow some steam to escape.

6. Allow the buns to cool for about 15 minutes before slicing them in half and serving.

Makes 12 buns.

English Muffins

You will need to have English muffin rings to make this gluten-free version of the traditional breakfast bread. These can be found in any cooking or kitchen store and are crucial to producing perfectly light English muffins. If you like your muffins more chewy, leave one egg out and use a little less milk.

- 1 cup warm water (110–115 degrees F)
- ½ cup almond milk (110–115 degrees F)
- 1 teaspoon granulated sugar
- 1 tablespoon active dry yeast
- 1 cup sorghum flour
- 1 cup tapioca starch
- ½ cup millet flour
- 2 teaspoons xanthan gum
- 1 teaspoon sea salt
- ¼ cup extra-virgin olive oil
- 2 tablespoons honey
- 2 large eggs

1. In a medium bowl, combine the water, almond milk, sugar, and yeast and stir. Set aside until the yeast gets foamy, about 10 minutes.

2. In a large bowl, stir together the sorghum flour, tapioca starch, millet flour, xanthan gum, and sea salt.

3. Add the yeast mixture to the dry ingredients along with the oil, honey, and eggs.

4. Mix the dough thoroughly and then allow the dough to rest for a few minutes.

5. Spoon the rested dough into eight English muffin rings placed on a baking sheet.

6. Place the baking sheet in a warm place, and allow the dough to rise until it is double in height.

7. Preheat oven to 350 degrees F.

8. Bake English muffins for about 20–25 minutes, until firm and a little golden.

9. Cool muffins on a wire rack and serve split open and toasted.

Makes 8 English muffins.

Sweet Potato Cornbread

This bread should be eaten warm with a steaming bowl of spicy chili. It is dense and slightly sweet, and it has a pretty rosy color due to the sweet potato. The sweet potato should be roasted very soft and mashed ahead of time. Make sure it is not too hot when you stir it into the batter, or the cornbread will end up slightly soggy and too heavy.

- 1 cup gluten-free, all-purpose flour
- 1 cup cornmeal
- ¼ cup granulated sugar
- 2 tablespoons gluten-free baking powder
- 1 teaspoon sea salt
- ½ teaspoon xanthan gum
- 3 large eggs, lightly beaten
- ½ cup sour cream
- 5 tablespoons melted coconut oil, plus extra to grease baking pan
- 2 tablespoons honey
- 2 large baked sweet potatoes, skin removed and mashed (about 1½ cups)

1. Preheat oven to 375 degrees F and lightly grease a 9-inch square baking pan.

2. In a large bowl, mix together the flour, cornmeal, sugar, baking powder, sea salt, and xanthan gum until well combined.

3. Add the eggs, sour cream, coconut oil, and honey, mixing well to combine after each addition.

4. Add the mashed sweet potatoes, and stir to combine. The batter will be thick at this point.

5. Spoon the batter into the prepared pan and smooth the top.

6. Bake for 40–50 minutes, until the top is golden brown and a knife inserted in the center comes out clean.

7. Allow the cornbread to cool at least 15 minutes, and then cut into squares. Serve warm.

Makes 8 servings.

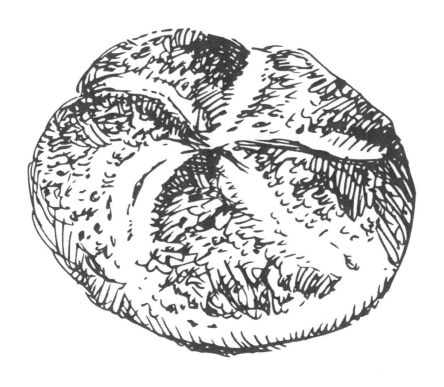

The smell of good bread baking, like the sound of lightly flowing water, is indescribable in its evocation of innocence and delight.

—M. F. K. Fisher

5

CELIAC DISEASE, WHEAT ALLERGY, AND GLUTEN SENSITIVITY

The reported number of patients diagnosed with some form of reaction to gluten is on the rise in Western countries. The reason for this increase is not fully understood. Some blame it on the high amounts of processed foods, breads, and baked goods in our diet. Another theory is that we are not exposed to enough antigens during childhood while our immune systems are developing, so our immune systems see gluten as an interloper or allergen.

Three main types of diagnoses are related to gluten reactions: celiac disease, wheat allergy, and gluten sensitivity. Since they share many symptoms, it's important to get a correct diagnosis from your doctor because a self-diagnosis based on your symptoms stands a decent chance of being incorrect and can lead to the wrong corrective action.

Celiac Disease

Celiac disease is considered the most serious of the three types of gluten reactions and is often misdiagnosed as irritable bowel syndrome or a food intolerance such as a wheat allergy. Often, it is only when treatment for these issues doesn't alleviate symptoms that doctors begin looking at celiac disease as a possibility.

If celiac disease is suspected, a doctor will order blood tests to detect and measure two types of antibodies: IgA-tTG (immunoglobulin A [IgA] anti-tissue transglutaminase [tTG] antibody) and IgA-EMA (immunoglobulin A [IgA] antiendomysial antibody [EMA]). If these antibodies are detected, doctors often confirm the diagnosis of celiac disease with a biopsy of the small intestine conducted during an endoscopy. An endoscopy is performed by guiding a small scope (called an endoscope) into the small intestine via the throat.

The small intestine is lined with microscopic projections that look a bit like sea anemone, called villi. The job of the villi is to absorb vitamins, fats, and other nutrients from foods as they pass through the small intestine. What's left is waste and moves on to the large intestine to be eliminated.

In a person with celiac disease, the villi flatten out and the lining of the small intestine becomes swollen or inflamed. This decreases the absorption of nutrients and can result in stunted growth, anemia, osteoporosis, and malnutrition. This inability to absorb nutrients is often what alerts doctors to celiac disease in children, as they fail to grow and gain weight at a normal rate.

One of the reasons celiac disease is underdiagnosed is that it produces a wide array of symptoms that can vary in incidence and severity. They include:

- abdominal swelling
- anemia
- bloating
- constipation
- diarrhea
- fatigue

- fatty stools
- frequent headaches
- gas
- nausea
- vomiting
- weight loss despite normal appetite

Because of the decreased absorption of nutrients, celiac disease can also result in depression, frequent respiratory infections, delayed puberty, trouble with memory or concentration, and irritability.

The treatment for celiac disease is a gluten-free diet, often accompanied by vitamin supplementation to correct common deficiencies. Many people with celiac disease tend to be deficient in fat-soluble vitamins such as A, D, K, and E. That's because in people with the disease, fat is poorly absorbed from the intestines. And when fat is not absorbed, the vitamins that dissolve in it are also not absorbed. Frequently, levels of calcium, iron, magnesium, zinc, folate, selenium, and copper are also low, for the same reason, and need to be supplemented.

Wheat Allergy

People with a wheat allergy may initially suspect they have celiac disease. This is a logical assumption, since the two problems share many common symptoms, and those symptoms are triggered by eating many of the same foods. Only proper testing can correctly identify the problem. The symptoms of a wheat allergy vary in intensity, based largely on the amount of wheat eaten. They include:

- anaphylaxis (swelling of the throat, difficulty breathing)
- cramps, nausea, vomiting, or any combination of these

- diarrhea
- hives, itchy rash, or swelling of the skin
- itchy, watery eyes
- nasal congestion
- swelling, itching, irritation of the mouth or throat, or any combination of these

In a person with a wheat allergy, the allergen is the wheat itself, not the gluten. This means people with a wheat allergy can't eat foods containing wheat and wheat flour, but unlike people with celiac disease, they can safely eat foods made with barley, rye, and oats. Wheat allergy is one of the most common food allergies found in children.

Some people with a wheat allergy choose to go on a gluten-free diet because it seems simpler and they feel it may be a healthier diet overall.

Gluten Sensitivity

Gluten sensitivity has only recently been recognized as a condition separate from celiac disease. Although the cause of gluten sensitivity is still being intensely researched, the medical community now agrees that it is a separate disorder.

There is no specific diagnostic test for gluten sensitivity. Your doctor will generally use your medical history and a physical examination combined with your own reporting of symptoms you experience when eating products made with or containing gluten. Doctors often rule out celiac disease first. Even if the key diagnostic antibodies are present, the villi and small intestine will not show the damage that occurs in people with celiac disease.

The symptoms of gluten sensitivity are often the same as those of celiac disease, although they may differ in severity or frequency. The most common symptoms include:

- fatigue
- frequent headaches
- gastrointestinal distress (particularly gas, bloating, and nausea)

Commonly, doctors advise a gluten-free diet for those with gluten sensitivity, although these patients will probably not require additional vitamin supplements, since they suffer some of the same reactions to gluten but not the villi damage that inhibits nutrient absorption.

Whether you've chosen to adopt a gluten-free diet because of celiac disease, wheat allergy, or gluten sensitivity, you can expect to feel a great deal better once you've been on a gluten-free diet for a short time. If you don't see a marked improvement in symptoms, it's extremely important to see your doctor to rule out any other conditions, such as Crohn's disease or irritable bowel syndrome.

Lactose Intolerance and Celiac Disease

Some people diagnosed with celiac disease also find that they are lactose intolerant. This is because of the damage done to the villi in the small intestine. The cells lining the small intestine produce an enzyme called lactase, which is necessary for digesting lactose, the sugar that occurs naturally in milk and milk products. The damage that causes celiac disease results in both a deficiency of lactase and the villi's inability to catch and break down lactose molecules.

If you've just been diagnosed with celiac disease, ask your doctor about testing you for lactose intolerance as well. Don't be discouraged about having to give up another food group. In many cases, the lactose intolerance is only temporary, and once the villi are able to repair themselves (within six months to a year after going gluten-free), you can often go back to eating dairy. However, lactose intolerance and its symptoms can continue for some time after you go on a gluten-free diet; sometimes, for as long as two years.

After you have been gluten-free for a year, ask your doctor to retest you for lactose intolerance. Your small intestine and villi may be healthy enough to produce sufficient lactase by this time. Until then, you can substitute almond milk, soy milk, or rice milk for drinking, cooking, and lightening your coffee. You can even find cheese, yogurt, and ice cream made from these dairy alternatives. The recipes in this book that contain dairy products can easily be changed to reflect a lactose-free version. Simply substitute the offending ingredient with a lactose-free product.

Were Our Bodies Designed to Eat Gluten?

The rising number of people diagnosed with celiac disease and gluten sensitivity has attracted more attention to the theory that our bodies are simply not genetically designed to eat grains. This theory is what has led to the popularity of the Paleolithic, Paleo, or Stone Age diet.

There are some scientific studies that support this theory. It's true that until about 10,000 years ago, grains were not cultivated and thus were not a part of the daily human diet. It's also true that people in pre-agricultural times did not seem to have suffered from the various metabolic and digestive disorders that have been attributed to eating grains and processed foods such as breads, cereals, pastries, and other modern favorites. The rate of metabolic syndrome, type 2 diabetes, obesity, and other such disorders has risen dramatically in the past few decades, and many nutritionists and researchers blame the fact that processed grains make up a growing proportion of the typical daily diet.

Researchers and nutritionists who have recommended removing grains and legumes from our diets suggest that our bodies have not had enough time to adapt genetically to absorbing and processing grains. Since gluten comes from grains, it may follow that we're not genetically adapted to eating it, either.

The jury is still out on whether eating grains is bad for our health. But quite a few people have chosen to follow diets like the Paleo diet, which is a gluten-free diet that is also very high in protein. Many people following the Paleo diet report better digestive health, more energy, and less inflammation.

Scientists can't confidently say that all grains are bad for your health. They do know that wheat, barley, rye, and possibly oats that contain gluten are dangerous for those with celiac disease and gluten sensitivity, and that wheat and wheat products are a health threat to those with a wheat allergy.

Is a Gluten-Free Diet Healthy for Everyone?

Obviously, a gluten-free diet is essential for those who have been diagnosed with either celiac disease or gluten sensitivity. It's also a simple option for those who have a wheat allergy, as it takes much of the guesswork and label reading out of the equation. But is going gluten-free beneficial to the rest of us? The answer is "maybe."

Researchers and scientists agree that humans have been eating grains only for less than 1 percent of our history as a species. There's still a good deal of debate about whether that fact has any significance when it comes to health and nutrition, but many well-respected nutritionists believe it does. Many followers of diets such as the Paleo diet agree, and they report feeling much better overall, with fewer digestive issues and headaches, and an increase in energy.

If you're going gluten-free because you think it might be healthier, or if you have a wheat allergy and are going gluten-free altogether, you'll likely be reducing the unhealthy fats, sugars, and preservatives that often come with flour-based foods.

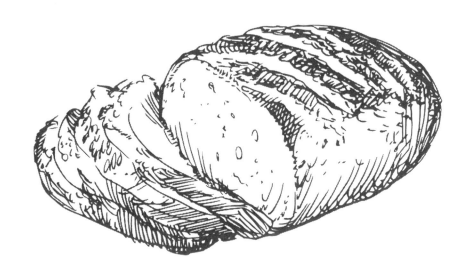

Bread is like dresses, hats, and shoes —in other words, essential!

—Emily Post

6

REAL-WORLD GLUTEN-FREE—HOW IT WORKS

Going on any diet requires some work. You have to plan, strategize, compromise, and commit. When your diet is required medically, there's the added stress of knowing you can't just quit when you get bored or frustrated. But for any diet to be successful, you have to be able to stick with it. The best diets:

- are as easy as possible to follow
- provide plenty of nutrition and variety
- give you ways to enjoy the foods you really love, such as bread and muffins
- are accessible and affordable for everyone
- are convenient

Real-world gluten-free living means being able to stick with your diet no matter how busy you are, or whether you're in a restaurant or your own home. It means you have to be able to feed yourself without going broke or feeling like your diet is a part-time job. It means knowing how to stick with your diet without feeling separate from everyone else. Gluten is in so many packaged products and comes in so many forms that going gluten-free also means reading food labels and becoming expert at finding hidden gluten.

Know How to Replace the Foods You Cannot Have

It's easy to get discouraged and upset when you think you can never again have cinnamon rolls, a blueberry muffin, or a hearty sandwich. Fortunately, going gluten-free in the real world means you can have your cake and eat it, too. The recipe collection here includes gluten-free ways to enjoy many of your favorite baked breads, rolls, and even pizza doughs that you probably thought you'd have to give up for good.

Have Plenty of Choices

Some of us love to cook and have plenty of time to spend doing it. Others are on very tight schedules or just don't enjoy spending much time in the kitchen. The recipe selection in this book will give you a wide array of breads that suit your needs and lifestyle. There are quick and easy treats you can throw together in a snap, as well as more involved recipes for those who love to bake breads from scratch.

Going gluten-free isn't necessarily simple, and it definitely isn't without compromise; however, it can also be delicious, affordable, and easier than you ever thought possible.

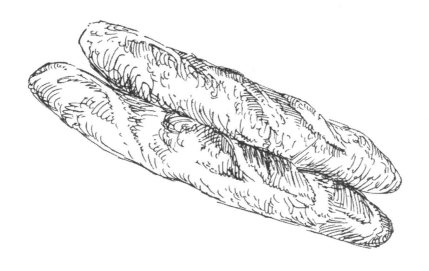

*Rather a piece of bread with a
happy heart than wealth with grief.*

—Egyptian Proverb

7

MAKING YOUR HOME GLUTEN-FREE

You can take several steps to make your home gluten-free and safe for you or someone else who has celiac disease or gluten sensitivity. It's not just a matter of getting rid of products you cannot eat—although that's a huge portion of the task. Obviously, if you are going on a gluten-free diet voluntarily, without medical orders, you can be more lenient about following these guidelines.

If all of this seems like it may be unnecessarily thorough, consider this information from Alexandra Anca, MHSc, RD, who cowrote *The Complete Gluten-Free Diet and Nutrition Guide*:

> We know that one-seventieth of a slice of bread causes intestinal damage in celiac disease. The question remains, what kind of damage does ingestion of a bread crumb cause? We don't know. If it happens daily or frequently, it will keep the inflammatory response active and the lining of the intestine will continue to be damaged. The more frequent the accidents, the less time in which your body has a chance to heal. This leads to complications and unresolved symptoms.

What llows is a list of the things you'll need to do to make your home gluten-free.

Get Rid of Gluten Products or Segregate Them

If you're going to make your entire kitchen gluten-free, bundle up all the products that contain gluten, including cereals, crackers, cookies, cakes, breads, and anything else that includes wheat, barley, or rye in the ingredients list. You can donate unopened packages to a food bank, local church, day-care center, or homeless shelter. Opened packages can be passed on to friends and family who will use them. As a last resort, throw opened items away.

If you have a family, partner, or roommate who will not be going gluten-free, you should at least segregate the gluten-free products from those containing gluten. If space is at a premium, you can get some storage jars or containers with tight lids in which to store your gluten-free products once they've been opened. This will protect them from cross-contamination.

Get a New Toaster

If you like toast, you'll need to buy a new toaster, since it's extremely difficult to clean an already-used toaster well enough to make it safe for someone with celiac disease. This is especially important if you have others in the home who will be toasting bread containing gluten. Label yours so that everyone knows it's the designated gluten-free toaster.

If you plan to eat toast on vacation, bring your toaster with you so you can toast your gluten-free bagels, bread, and waffles. You won't be able to use the toaster that's provided in your room, vacation property, or hotel's self-serve dining area.

Buy New Jars of Condiments

Any opened condiments in your refrigerator or cabinets have most likely been contaminated with gluten crumbs, so buy a new supply of condiments, including jam and jellies, mustard, ketchup, peanut butter, margarine, mayonnaise, and anything else you enjoy using on your breads. Label your jars so other household members know to leave them alone.

Replace Plastic Items and Nonstick Pans

Plastic bowls and utensils scratch easily, allowing tiny amounts of gluten to become embedded in the surface. The same is true of nonstick pots and pans. You'll need to replace these or get a second set for gluten-free cooking. Try to get brightly colored pans that are clearly separate from what you already have, so that they're not mistakenly used to prepare foods containing gluten.

It's safe to use stainless steel or glass pans and bowls for both gluten and gluten-free foods, as long as you wash them carefully.

Have Separate Equipment for Gluten-Free Flours

There's no way you can clean all the nooks and crannies in a flour sifter, so just buy yourself a new one and keep it in a separate spot in the kitchen. And remember, handling wheat flour in a kitchen used to prepare gluten-free food is dangerous, as wheat flour can stay airborne for hours. If you must sift wheat flour, cover or remove all gluten-free food from the area.

Unless you are able to wash it in a dishwasher, you will definitely need to buy a new colander or strainer. Those tiny holes are almost impossible to clean thoroughly by hand.

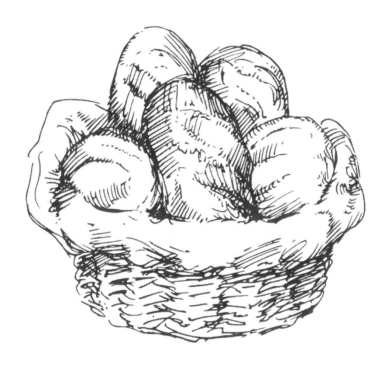

Without bread, all is misery.

—William Cobbett

8

THE BEST SUBSTITUTES FOR WHEAT, RYE, AND BARLEY FLOURS

For people who can't have gluten, baked goods are often a source of disappointment instead of the enjoyable indulgence they are meant to be. The typical flours used for baking and cooking include rye, barley, and wheat flours, all of which have at least a small amount of gluten. Fortunately, there are several good flour alternatives you can use to turn that bread or pastry into a delicious, gluten-free treat that even your family will enjoy.

Good Gluten-Free Flours for Baking

Because different flours interact differently with the other ingredients in a recipe, some gluten-free flours are more suited to baking than others. If you're making a cake, pizza dough, or pastry, the best flours to use include rice flour, sorghum flour, tapioca flour, and potato flour. Remember to add xanthan gum (or guar gum) so you get a good rise and a nice texture.

It's best if you experiment and find your own preferred blends, but when you substitute flours in your favorite traditional recipes, use the following measurements per cup of wheat flour.

Rice flour: Substitute ¾ cup for every 1 cup wheat flour, 1¼ cups barley flour, or 1⅓ cups rye flour. If you use rice flour, be aware that your baked product may have a grainy texture. Since this is one of the more readily available gluten-free flours, you may choose to accept the textural issues in favor of convenience. If possible, mix in ¼ cup of either potato or tapioca flour per cup of rice flour to improve the texture. You can also try brown rice flour, which is harder to find and a little more expensive, but also less grainy.

Tapioca flour: Substitute tapioca cup for cup with wheat flour. Use 1 cup tapioca for every 1¼ cups barley flour or 1⅓ cups rye flour.

Potato flour: Substitute ¾ cup potato flour for every 1 cup wheat flour, every 1¼ cups barley flour, or every 1⅓ cups rye flour. This is because potato flour is a bit heavier. Also, if you use potato flour, remember that it tastes like potato and may change the flavor of your recipe. If you're concerned about this, try mixing it with tapioca or rice flour.

Sorghum flour: Perhaps the best-tasting flour, this should be used in equal amounts when substituting for wheat, rye, or barley flours.

Good Gluten-Free Substitutes for Batter

If you want to batter fish, meats, or vegetables to fry or bake them, some good substitutions include corn flour or rice flour mixed with ¼ teaspoon gluten-free baking powder. Don't use guar gum or xanthan gum for batters; it's not necessary.

Good Gluten-Free Substitutions for Pancakes

Just about everybody loves pancakes, crepes, and waffles for breakfast, but people who need to go gluten-free usually have to skip them. Well, now you don't have to do that! Just substitute rice, sorghum, or buckwheat flour in your pancake, crepe, and waffle recipes.

Buckwheat flour is naturally gluten-free, but remember that it has a very distinctive flavor and texture. Also, make sure that when you buy it, it actually says "gluten-free," because buckwheat flour is frequently processed with the same machinery that processes wheat flour and may become contaminated. If you're making pancakes, crepes, or waffles, you want them to rise, so remember to use xanthan gum or guar gum in your batter, regardless of which gluten-free flour you're using.

Choosing the Best Gluten-Free Flour for the Job

Here are some good basic rules to use when trying to decide which flour to use:

- Medium gluten-free flours, such as brown rice flour and sorghum flour, are similar to using white, all-purpose flour.

- Heavier gluten-free grain flours, such as buckwheat, millet, cornmeal, and legume or bean flours, are similar to baking with whole-grain flours such as barley and rye.

When it comes right down to it, your choice of gluten-free flour substitutions is all about what tastes good to you. Experiment—try mixing the different flours and figure out what works best for your particular tastes. The fact that you can't have gluten doesn't mean you have to go without bread or batter-fried foods. Also, several of the top prepackaged cake and dessert manufacturers now offer gluten-free options that taste great and are just as convenient to make as their gluten-containing cousins. Whatever you do though, don't think your pizza and muffin days are over just because you can't have gluten.

INDEX

Lightning Source UK Ltd.
Milton Keynes UK
UKOW03f2333091213

222687UK00014B/319/P